# Healthy Meals in Minutes

Tracy Dwyer

Published by FastPencil Publishing

Healthy Meals in Minutes

First Edition

Print edition ISBN: 9781499905243



http://www.fastpencil.com

Printed in the United States of America

# TABLE OF CONTENTS

# Chapter 1: My Reasons for Writing Healthy Meals in Minutes

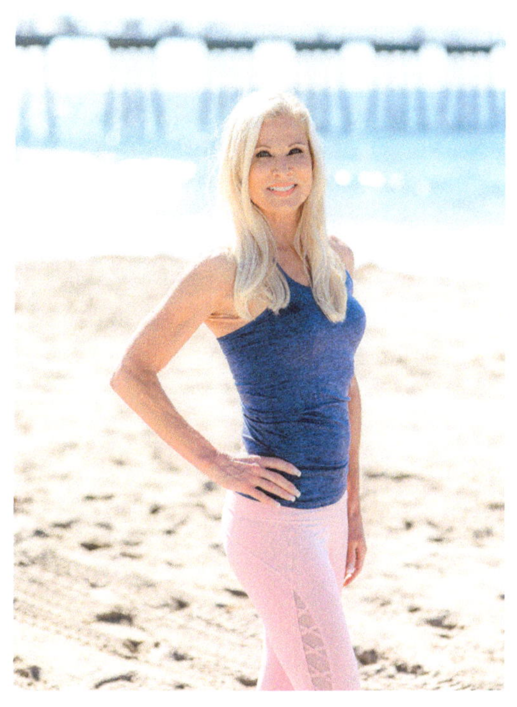

This is not just another book about how to eat healthy. It is a book about how to *live* a healthy lifestyle and improve your life through healthy eating and exercise. Learning to create nutritious meals quickly and schedule time to exercise will give you more energy and more time to focus on your goals in life. When you make health your priority it creates a new outlook on life. This reduces stress and creates a world of opportunities.

Over the years I have been asked how I stay in shape and what I eat. I have a Bachelor of Arts degree from Loyola Marymount in Film and Television which made writing a book a logical way to share my secrets with the world. Helping others has always been a top priority for me, and through a book I can reach many people and share what I do to stay healthy and fit.

Many people think it takes too much time and costs too much money to eat healthy. In reality it is more about time management, planning your meals, and taking time to exercise. I will teach you how to make healthy food choices, navigate the grocery store, and create great tasting meals in minutes.

Everyone wants to be healthy, but there is a lot of confusing information on television and online which leaves people feeling like it is too hard to do. They will stick with poor food choices because they don't want to look for creditable information or go on a diet. Obesity has become an epidemic in this country contributing to diseases such as type 2 diabetes, high cholesterol, high blood pressure, heart disease, and more. These diseases are even being seen in children. One in three children are obese and many of them already have illnesses that could have been prevented by eating healthy foods.

My goal is to teach you how to follow my healthy eating plan and make your life healthier and happier. Teaching your children to eat healthy will help them make wise food choices throughout their lives. Living a healthy lifestyle includes eating nutritious foods and getting daily exercise. This in turn greatly reduces your chances of getting a life-threatening disease.

By learning how to take care of yourself and to make healthy meals in minutes you will have more time in the day for things you enjoy. The ease of creating a shopping list and navigating the grocery store will keep you from running to the store every day and will make eating fast food and junk food a thing of the past.

Once you make healthy eating a habit and see the great results that come from it, you will never go back to eating unhealthy foods again. Right now is a great time to start eating healthy and have your family enjoying healthy delicious meals.

It was a natural for me to write this book. Life has not always been easy for me, but along the way I learned so much about health, nutrition, exercise, stress, and overcoming disease. Although I started out with a full scholarship to Pepperdine University to become a doctor, life took many twists and turns. In the end, I never became a doctor, but my desire to help people with their health and fitness remains to this day.

Life taught me much about everything from responsibility to raising children, from being financially responsible as a single mom to living in optimum health in the face of life-changing disease. This book is not a collection of mere good ideas, facts, and figures. It shares with you the lifestyle I have lived for more than two decades and continue to live today.

The life-changing disease I mentioned challenged me when I was 36 years old. At that time I was diagnosed with colon cancer. I was the youngest person the doctors had seen with it. I was scheduled to have major surgery in a month. I was not going to let the diagnosis of cancer get me down. I had to take action and do whatever I could to beat it. I started reading books on nutrition and learning which foods help fight cancer.

I went on a vegetarian diet that was 100% organic. Every day I ate a lot of fresh vegetables and fruits and drank green drinks made with spinach, parsley, carrots, celery, and greens. I got my body as strong as I could, and I took the time to be grateful and pray for a full recovery. I asked everyone I knew to put me on their prayer list at church.

Going to the gym had already become a part of my daily routine, but now it was a necessity to get my body as strong as possible and ready for surgery. I needed to do everything I could to insure a full recovery from the surgery and to rid myself of cancer. Aerobics classes and weight lifting helped reduce my stress and get my body strong.

To make a very long story short (it's going to be another book), the surgery was successful, the cancer was completely gone, and my 8-week recovery was a complete success. Though I didn't realize it at the time, this whole process of overcoming colon cancer was the start of my healthy eating plan—the same plan I'm sharing with you in this book!

My strength and determination come from my will to remain healthy and to live a long active life. My healthy eating plan and daily exercise have made me the picture of health and an inspiration to others.

Whether you are trying to eat healthier, lose weight, or improve your fitness level, this healthy meal plan will work for you. Remember, this is not a diet. You don't have to eliminate food groups, count points, or count calories! Using my plan, you will create healthy meals in minutes.

This is an eating plan and so much more. It is truly a lifestyle plan. Because of that, I will also teach you how to deal with food and exercise in those challenging times we all face in life, such as when you travel, when you eat out, or when your schedule is crowded by all the responsibilities of family, work, and life in general. This book will equip you with all the information you will need to create the healthy life that you and your family deserve.

# CHAPTER 2: WHAT IS HEALTHY EATING?

Everything you put into your body has a profound effect on it. When you give your body the right type of food, you will feel great, look great, and have more energy. Fruits, vegetables, beans, legumes, 100% whole grains, lean proteins, and healthy fats are all needed for your body to function properly and run strong.

Think about your body as if it were a nice car. Most people take great care of their car on the inside by putting the right gas in the tank and getting the oil changed on a regular basis. Then they take it to the car wash and make it look good on the outside. Taking care of the car is a priority because you use it to get to work, pick up your kids, and as a way to get everywhere you need to go.

In much the same way, your body is working around the clock to keep you going throughout your day and repairing itself at night while you sleep. Shouldn't you take great care of your body also? Indeed, your health should be the most important thing in your life. Taking care of "you" is more important than anything else. If you do not take care of yourself, how can you take care of your family or help anyone else?

When you are in an airliner there are instructions in the seat-back pocket. Those instructions are given before each flight by the flight attendants. They say that if the cabin loses pressure the oxygen mask will come down. Put your own mask on first and then help children and others. Why? This is because if you do not help yourself first, you won't be able to help anyone else.

Keep this in mind when you think about your health and what is important in life. When people are facing illnesses, or are on their deathbed they never say they wish they had eaten more junk food or watched more television. They say they wish they had taken better care of themselves. Remember to take care of YOU.

## YOU ARE WHAT YOU EAT, SO EAT HEALTHY!

In many of my motivational speeches I say, "You are what you eat, so why would you eat a greasy hamburger or fried foods?" When it comes to what foods are bad for you, there's a good chance that you do know what you should avoid eating. It is clear that fried foods, sugary drinks, and junk foods are not good for you.

Eating healthy is about eating foods in their natural state when possible and when cooked, prepared without batter, butter, greasy sauces, or sugary toppings. There are so many options in the world of healthy foods. It is not boring to eat healthy when you know what your options are and how to prepare your foods to make them healthy and taste good.

Learning to love the taste of whole foods in their natural state is a great way to improve your health. Fruits and vegetables are loaded with vitamins and fiber that are necessary to maintain good health.

Food should never be used as a reward or a punishment because it creates an unhealthy relationship with food. This does not mean you can never let yourself or your kids have a cookie or a piece of cake. Just don't use it as a reward or take it away as a punishment. Doing this can put some strong negatives into play.

## THE POWER OF POSITIVE THINKING

You might be asking yourself, *what is this section doing in a chapter about healthy eating?* and it is a great question! The short answer is *it has everything to do with it.* While it is true that healthy eating is about food choices and learning what is good for you and what is not, there is a deeper side to it as well.

Once you learn what is healthy and what is not, how do you make those decisions to change? How do you stick with your newfound healthy lifestyle? To a very great degree, your success depends on your ability to coach yourself day by day. That is where positivity comes into play in a very big way, and that's why I placed this section in this chapter for you.

There is nothing quite as powerful or effective as positive thinking and positive self-talk when it comes to bringing changes to your life. What you think and what you say have a profound effect on how you feel, what you achieve, and even on what you eat.

When you are positive about the changes you are making, they become very simple. When negative thoughts enter the mind, they block productivity and can even bring about failure. Whether you are starting to eat healthy and exercise, running a race, or interviewing for a new job, it is important to always be positive.

I have had a lot of unexpected challenges happen in my life. School, marriage, divorce, being a single mom, career changes, colon cancer, emotional upheavals and countless other things have shown up through the years to derail me if they could. However, I managed to make it successfully through everything that came my way. How? By keeping my thoughts and my self-talk positive.

When the colon cancer was diagnosed, along with eating organic and exercising, part of my plan was to use the power of positive thinking to get me through both the surgery and recovery. I am living proof that it worked! I read motivational books, listened to motivational speakers, and used visualization and mantras all day, every day. I asked everyone to pray for me and I prayed for myself. After five days in the hospital I was told the cancer had not spread and I would not need any further treatment.

Once the recovery period was behind me, I began thinking about starting a new business. Once again, I used the power of positive thinking and went on to create a successful traveling notary service.

After doing that for some time I decided I wanted to become an actor. Again I used visualization and mantras, and again, I was successful. I became an actor on television series including *Nash Bridges*. I was also in a movie, *Patch Adams*, and got to meet the real Patch Adams and Robin Williams. I was also in many local and national commercials.

Using positive thinking is very important in the quest for anything you want to do in your life. Whether you need to start eating healthy or just improve on your eating habits, having a positive outlook will help you succeed.

Positive self-talk is as important as positive thinking and is vital to good health. If you are constantly telling yourself that you can't do something or saying anything negative to yourself, it lowers your self-esteem and can cause you to fail. It's not because you are unable to achieve your goal. It is because you are planting doubt in your mind.

Think about what you say to yourself. Many people say things to themselves that they would never say to anyone else. Positive self-talk and being your own cheerleader are necessary. Make speaking positive at all times a priority, especially when you are talking to yourself. No matter what happens, pat yourself on the back for having a great day and making positive changes. Don't wait for approval from others. Give approval to yourself and visualize yourself as the successful person you can be and you will be.

## TAKE ACTION!

Taking action is required for the implementation of any plan, so do something right away and you will feel like you are moving in the right direction. Eliminate fast foods, processed foods, sugary snacks, and fatty foods. Make up your mind today to eat healthy for yourself and for your family.

It is human nature for people to want to gain pleasure from what they do and to get out of any type of pain. This is a driving factor in many decisions that you make. If you look at your positive changes as being more pleasurable for you than continuing your bad habits, your brain will derive pleasure from your new way of doing things. When you give more pleasure to eating an apple than to eating a piece of candy you will feel pleasure in eating the apple and won't miss the candy. This is especially true when you see the changes in your body. Eating healthy foods will help you lose weight and exercise will help you put on muscle and get stronger. All these positive changes will happen rapidly when you are eating healthy all the time and loving what you eat.

This meal plan is very easy and any of the meals can be eaten for breakfast, lunch, or dinner. If you aren't hungry in the morning, eat a snack and have a mid-morning breakfast followed by lunch. If you have a busy schedule and cannot eat three meals a day and two or three snacks, then combine some of your meals. By eating three meals a day with two or three snacks and getting daily exercise you keep your metabolism running and burning calories.

The more active you are the more calories you can consume. Your activity level will determine how much you can eat. I will give you guidelines and you can add foods when your activity level increases. If you are trying to lose weight and the weight is not coming off, increase your exercise or reduce your calories. Consult a doctor if you have any medical conditions.

If you are overweight, it will be very easy to lose the first 20-30 pounds just by cutting out the fast foods, processed foods, and alcohol which all contain a lot of calories and little nutrition. People who consume a lot of alcohol or drugs, or who have any medical conditions should consult a doctor before they stop drinking or using drugs as I am not a doctor. I can suggest that you start eating healthy foods all the time which helps reduce weight and provides the nutrients your body needs.

Using this healthy eating plan while you are eliminating alcohol or other addictions will help keep you from replacing them with overeating or other unwanted habits. Making it more pleasurable to eat healthy than to do things that are not healthy will give you a good outlook while making changes. Healthy eating will give your body the nutrients it needs. By using my healthy meal plan and getting daily exercise you can avoid the temptation to eat sugary snacks or use tobacco to replace another bad habit that you are trying to stop. By giving your body the nutrients it needs and munching on raw celery and carrots and eating a lot of fruits and vegetables you can eliminate cravings for things that are not healthy. Eating a healthy diet will improve your chances for success.

## PLAN YOUR MEALS

Planning is a major part of eating healthy. Without planning ahead, you won't make the healthiest food choices. I will teach you how to plan a variety of meals with vegetables and different types of protein. The key is in making several types of protein and steamed vegetables one or two days a week. Cooking enough for several meals at one time makes meals quick and easy to prepare.

I see many families struggle with trying to decide at the last minute what to eat for dinner. They have frozen chicken or fish in the freezer which takes time to thaw out. Or they may only have frozen junk foods that are breaded, fried, and full of artificial ingredients, sodium, fat, and calories.

Lack of planning makes ordering a pizza or running out for fast food seem like the easiest choice. But making that fast food run is never the healthy choice. Planning is needed. By planning ahead and stocking up on healthy foods in your refrigerator, freezer, and pantry, you create a lot of options for your meal planning and I will teach you how to use them all.

I used to come home from work on a cold afternoon and heat up tomato juice and frozen vegetables for a quick easy soup. The possibilities are endless when you have a variety of foods in your kitchen.

Another simple example can be taken from my life when I travel. I try to use up all the perishable foods before I leave so when I come home I don't have to go through the refrigerator and throw things away that have spoiled. When I get home from a three-week trip I don't have any food in the refrigerator, so I take something out of the freezer.

If I have white fish or a piece of thin fish, it will defrost quickly. I can also use a veggie patty or something that is already cooked and frozen. Turkey patties thaw out quickly and can be wrapped in a wet paper towel and defrosted in the microwave in just a minute or two. I have frozen vegetables so I can eat them with my patty. I also can use frozen shrimp and frozen mixed vegetables (Chinese and Thai vegetables taste great together) to make a stir "unfry" within minutes. I just put a little water in the pan, add the vegetables, and cook. I rinse cooked shrimp and add it to the vegetables and cook until hot. I like to add Bragg's Liquid Amino Acids instead of soy sauce. It has less sodium and tastes great. This can also be made with a little bit of sesame oil or sunflower oil, about a teaspoon is plenty. Brown rice or rice noodles can also be added to this for more nutrients.

With simple planning, stocking, and preparation, you, too, eliminate that thought of running out for fast food or even eating out in a restaurant. No matter what your circumstances or your schedule, you'll feel in control of your food and your health because you always have nutritious and quick cooking options at hand.

Nothing in life has any meaning other than what you give it. By making healthy eating an important part of your day you will understand the meaning of living a healthy lifestyle. It will be clear that what you need to do is focus on being healthy all year long. My plan is about making healthy attachments to healthy things. Knowing this will enhance your life and strengthen your convictions to living healthy.

# CHAPTER 3: HOW TO PLAN MEALS

Everything in life is simpler when you plan ahead. Healthy meals are easy to prepare when you plan ahead and have everything you need to make a meal in minutes. When you don't have to run to the store to buy food or go out for fast food it saves a lot of time and money. Planning and being organized takes the stress out of preparing meals.

My healthy eating plan is designed to make it easy for you to prepare nutritious, great tasting meals. It won't take long for you to learn how to create your own healthy meals using my plan. You can decide what foods to have for breakfast and which to have for lunch and dinner. If you feel like having eggs for dinner and a turkey burger for breakfast, that is perfectly fine. Just change the meals around.

If you are trying to lose weight, skip starchy carbohydrates at night. Unless you are an athlete or doing moderate to strenuous exercise every day, you don't need to eat starchy foods at night. Some people sleep better when they eat some carbohydrates with their evening meal. Choose nutrient dense carbohydrates like yams, squash, or even an ear of corn.

Don't worry about giving your children starchy carbohydrates at night. Make sure they are getting a good amount of vegetables in a wide variety along with their healthy protein so they will sleep well and have energy in the morning. If your child is overweight consult a pediatrician and/or a registered dietician who deals with overweight children. Cut out all junk food, sodas (even diet), fatty foods, and fast foods. Create healthy meals at home and prepare lunch for your child to take to school. Don't expect the school to prepare healthy foods or to focus on what your child is eating. They are serving whatever they are given to serve and it is highly processed and has a lot of preservatives so it will stay fresh for a long time. Cut down on pasta and make sure when you buy pasta that it is made with a 100% whole grain or is a vegetable pasta. Avoid all white flour products and make more yams, squash, salads, and vegetables.

The most important thing to remember is that we all have only one body and it is up to each one of us to take great care of it. Children need our help to guide them to eat healthy foods and avoid the sugary and processed foods. By giving our bodies the healthy foods it needs we will be healthy, happy, and have a lot of energy to use for doing things we enjoy.

## THE SHOPPING LIST

Making a shopping list is a very important part of learning how to eat healthy. The shopping list will help you buy nutritious foods while avoiding processed foods and sugar-filled items. Creating the list before you go to the store saves you time and money.

There are some items that you will always keep in the pantry or freezer and other things like milk, yogurt, eggs, and fresh fruits and vegetables that you will buy weekly. Don't worry about buying more fruit than you need because you can always freeze it and use it for a smoothie or frozen yogurt. When you have leftover vegetables make a stew or soup with all the vegetables and freeze what you will not use.

Plan on shopping in the morning or early afternoon instead of noon or 6:00 p.m. when stores are crowded. By keeping your shelves stocked with canned beans, tuna, 100% whole grain pasta, and organic tomato sauce or chunky canned tomatoes along with food in the freezer you should only need to go shopping one time per week. Use the foods you have at home and be creative when preparing your meals with leftovers. This will save time and money because you won't be running to the store all of the time.

When shopping, stay on the perimeter of the store to avoid the sugary snacks and processed food aisles. Many stores have an organic section in the produce aisle, organic cereal and cereal with low sugar in the cereal aisle and some mixed in with regular products. When you go to a new store ask one of the store employees where the organic section is so you aren't wandering around looking for what you need. Going up and down every aisle makes it very tempting to buy things that aren't healthy and that you do not need. This is especially true if you are hungry when shopping or have children with you.

Plan your meals in your head or write them down. When writing your shopping list, visualize the layout of your store. Write down the items you need in the order you come to them in the store. (There is more information about your shopping list in chapter seven.)

## ESSENTIAL FOODS TO KEEP ON HAND

I stock up on boneless chicken breasts, ahi tuna, and other fresh fish. Buy a variety of fresh fruits and vegetables to insure eating a wide variety of nutrients. Think about buying a variety of colors when choosing produce. There is always a big bowl of fresh fruits on my counter and many different types of vegetables in my refrigerator along with unsweetened almond milk, low- or non-fat milk, eggs, yogurt, and other items that can be turned into a quick healthy meal in minutes.

Take advantage of frozen foods as well. Ezekiel bread and Alvarado Street bread are both flourless breads that taste great and are very healthy. Both brands also have tortilla shells which are a great option for adding variety to your meals. You will also find a great selection of organic frozen vegetables. There are also some items I love to use for a quick healthy meal like Amy's Burritos. I like the bean and rice and the black bean and vegetable which do not have any cheese. These are helpful additions to have on hand all the time. The brown rice bowls are great to have in the freezer when you come home from a trip so you don't have to go to the store on your way home. There are other healthy options that you can explore in the frozen section. Freezing leftovers from meals you cook is always helpful because it does not take long to thaw something out for dinner. In the times it takes to unpack your suitcase, leftovers can be thawed out and ready to heat and eat.

Some stores sell previously frozen fish. There should be a sign or label that says it is previously frozen. Make sure to cook this fish within a day or two. It is fine to freeze fish, chicken, and beef after it is cooked. Make sure to freeze them within a few days and to eat them within two days of being thawed again. When you thaw fish, chicken, or other meat, remember to do so by placing it into the refrigerator. Never let it thaw on the countertop.

Keep some canned, organic, low-fat, refried beans, black beans, garbanzo beans, and kidney beans in your pantry. Have a variety of dried goods on your shelves also. Brown rice, organic thick-cut or steel-cut oatmeal, and quinoa are good choices that I always have in the pantry. Quinoa has all nine essential amino acids which make it a complete protein. Beans and rice make a complete protein and are low in fat and calories. They also add great flavor to any salad and can replace meat in any meal which makes them a perfect vegetarian option.

One thing you can do with fish, chicken, or beef is cook it and then freeze it. This way it does not go bad, and you will have cooked protein available for any meal. All you have to do is thaw your frozen food in a bowl of cold water and then heat it up. (See chapter seven for much more information including the complete list of foods that I use.)

## How to Begin My Healthy Eating Plan

At the beginning of each week, make a list of things to cook for the week. It is helpful to come up with several dishes you can make using each protein source. For example, you can buy several pounds of ground turkey breast, then use half of it for patties and half of it for chopped meat that can then be used in several dishes. Cook several chicken breasts and several types of fish that will create various meals over a few days. The size of your family and the type of meals you want to prepare will determine how much you cook in advance.

Eating organic is the best way to eliminate pesticides, herbicides, antibiotics, and hormones from your food. It may cost a few cents more per pound, but you will be saving a lot of money by not eating fast foods or eating at restaurants all of the time. Find ways to save money like making your coffee at home and not stopping for sugary snacks that aren't good for you anyway. Saving money on unnecessary things and spending it on healthy foods is one of the most important things you can do for your health. Take advantage of farmers markets and buy fresh produce. Make this a family affair. Take the kids and teach them how to pick out fruits and vegetables. Children love to help and farmers markets are kid-friendly.

Buy organic chicken and always buy organic beef. I recommend that you limit the amount of beef you eat and use the leanest cuts. You might want to substitute ground turkey breast for ground beef. Ground turkey breast is low in fat, so it is leaner than ground beef and has fewer calories. Many packages which say organic ground turkey breast have some dark meat and have more fat. Ground turkey breast is usually 99% fat free and contains just turkey breast which makes them leaner. By adding some Agave or organic ketchup or tamari soy sauce to the ground turkey before you cook it will add more moisture. Bragg's Liquid Amino Acids is also good for adding moisture. If you use soy or Bragg's Liquid Amino Acids you won't need to add salt.

Ground turkey really does taste great, and adding any type of salt-free seasoning or garlic powder gives it a nice taste. I also like to add some organic Agave ketchup or salsa to give the meat more moisture for certain dishes. Many times, I will just use garlic powder. There are all sorts of tricks to use and a variety of seasonings that you can use to give ground turkey breast more flavor. Experiment for yourself. You'll discover what you and your family like, and you'll be eating healthier, too.

Steam several types of non-starchy vegetables and some starchy vegetables like Japanese yams, some garnet or jewel yams, string beans and squash. Kabocha squash is my favorite. Make a pot of brown rice, quinoa, or other 100% whole grains. From these things that are already prepared you can make a variety of dishes during the week for lunch and dinner. They can also be eaten for breakfast the next morning. Having food cooked in advance will make preparing healthy meals very quick and easy.

Reheating the protein in a pan on top of the stove or in a steamer is better than using a microwave which usually dries out fish and poultry. If you must use the microwave, wrap the protein in a wet paper towel and cook it a few seconds at a time.

## SIMPLE COOKING TIPS

Everything can be cooked in a non-stick frying pan, on the stovetop, on a grill, a baking sheet, a steamer pot or steamer basket, in the oven, or in a microwave. If you don't have a non-stick pan use a little olive oil in the pan or olive oil cooking spray.

When you cook at home it is fine to use high-quality unsaturated oil such as olive oil in your dishes as long as you use it sparingly. Keep in mind that fat contains almost twice the calories per gram than carbohydrates have. Fat is needed by your body, but only in a very small amount.

The serving size of fat or oil is the size of the end of your thumb. Instead of just pouring oil into a pan, use a measuring spoon. Try to cut down the amount of oil you use or don't use any oil at all. Use as little oil as possible in order to cut down calories. When baking, you can even substitute applesauce for the oil.

Many dishes will taste the same or even better using less oil. Things like omitting butter and oil from your meals can cut down on the amount of calories you consume. If you don't use oil, make sure that you eat enough fatty fish in your diet to get the amount of fat your body needs. There are many other ways of getting the healthy fats that your body needs without using butter.

Other sources of healthy fat come from various foods. Avocados are a good healthy fat. Almonds, walnuts, olives, olive oil, ground flaxseeds, and fatty fish (salmon, mackerel, albacore tuna, lake trout, and herring) are high in omega 3 fatty acids.

Shortcuts to making healthy meals are always helpful and I use them many times. For example,

I steam a lot of vegetables at one time, then store them in Tupperware so they are ready to use in whatever dish I am making. When you are pressed for time and need to make a quick meal, it is important to have healthy options readily available. It is also a great idea to have healthy snacks in ready-to-go baggies or Tupperware so you can grab them on the run. Measure out a serving size of raw trail mix and make sure it is not the new type that has candy added to it. Create your own trail mix with raw mixed nuts, seeds, and some dried fruits. Put chopped carrots, celery, grapes, cherries or apples in serving size bags so they are ready to eat whenever you or the kids get hungry. If you have bags of chips in the pantry, which is the first place you will go. Get out of the habit of eating chips and get into the habit of eating real food. Eating brown rice cakes is a great option to eating chips and kids love them. The crunch is very satisfying and they come in a lightly salted option for those who want to or need to limit salt intake.

If you have a lot of vegetables left over, make a stir "unfry" to use up all the vegetables before they go bad or if you are going out of town. If you don't have enough fresh vegetables, use a bag of frozen Chinese, Thai, or other mixed vegetables. Place them in a wok or large frying pan with a little water or olive oil (even non-stick spray), and cook them until they are partially thawed.

Once thawing begins, add the steamed vegetables that are left over and heat them until all the vegetables are cooked. Add shelled edamame, lima beans, kidney beans, garbanzo beans, or tofu for a quick easy meal. Don't be worried about mixing frozen and steamed vegetables together. Just make sure the frozen vegetables are warmed through and the steamed vegetables are warm. If you are worried about it, you can cook them in two different frying pans then add them together.

Another way to make meals faster is to cook a few different types of protein or use firm tofu for your meals and mix your steamed vegetables with the protein. Wash and chop vegetables and keep them in Tupperware, adding them to your meals. You can also lightly steam them and eat them on the side.

Vegetables are always great with brown rice or quinoa, and adding beans makes a complete protein that you can use instead of using chicken, fish, or meat to complete your meal. Add egg to your cooked brown rice and vegetables to make "un-fried" rice. Just put a little non-stick spray or water in the frying pan to keep the rice from sticking and add Bragg's Liquid Amino Acids, Tamari soy sauce (both are gluten free), or light soy sauce.

Once you decide what meals you want for the week, take one day in the week to cook several types of protein and steam a variety of starchy and non-starchy vegetables. Prepare enough protein and vegetable options to cover meals for the week such as chicken breast, ground turkey breast patties, ground turkey breast chopped into crumbles to use for salads, burritos, tostadas, breakfast salads, spaghetti sauce, and tacos. Chicken breast can also be substituted instead of ground turkey breast. Tofu does not need to be prepared in advance. It can be kept in the refrigerator and used for any dish. Tofu does have an expiration date on the package so be sure to use it before it expires.

Everything that takes time to cook, such as brown rice, quinoa, yams, or winter squash can be cooked and stored in the refrigerator. They can be used in many dishes or as a snack. I love to eat half of a Japanese or Garnet yam for a snack. I also love my kabocha squash with mashed cauliflower and mixed vegetables. The mixed vegetables can be from a frozen package or fresh. Heat them up and add them to the squash and cauliflower for a nutrient-packed snack or with a meal.

Cooking foods ahead of time makes healthy eating an easy choice. Meals become simple to put together because you planned and prepared ahead of time. While it can be fun to make a big meal for a special occasion, on a day-to-day basis it is too time consuming for most of us. Keeping meals simple is the key to having the ability to create healthy meals in minutes. By having a number of options in the refrigerator and freezer you do not have to stick with the first meal you plan to cook. If you change your mind it only takes a matter of minutes to make another dish and serve it instead.

Planning meals is also the best way to maintain your blood sugar level and to avoid eating foods that are not healthy. Low nutrition, excess fat, sodium, sugar and artificial ingredients are found in things like colas, doughnuts, and junk foods, fast foods, and processed foods. Avoiding these can cut a lot of unnecessary calories and harmful chemicals from every meal and snack.

This healthy eating plan is a way of life and a way to live a long life. It is not a diet. It is something that you will be able to live with and stick with. By making healthy eating a priority you will make healthy choices a natural habit. This can also free you from yo-yo dieting which makes your weight go up and down. Eating healthy will put you in a healthy state of mind and lead you to do everything that is good for you and avoid what is bad for you.

For the most part, people know what they should and should not eat. Eating an apple is better than eating a doughnut or a candy bar. Making healthy foods available by having them in your home helps you and your family know what to eat. When your shelves are stocked with healthy food choices it will create an anchor in your mind that these are the foods you will choose when you are hungry.

## FAST FOOD NATION

When fast foods became available our society became a fast food nation. People thought they could get a burger that was already prepared faster than they could cook one at home. Chains of fast food restaurants started to grow in massive numbers.

Fast food is now available anytime of the day or night. People are getting fatter in America and new fast food restaurants open every day. Eating fast food will cause weight gain. If you have to get fast food while on a long trip and nothing else is available, make sure to choose wisely. In the quest to keep customers coming to fast food restaurants free toys are given with a children's meal which makes kids beg to go get a fast meal with a free prize. My suggestion is to make them a turkey burger at home and buy them a toy.

There are some health-conscious foods at some fast food restaurants like a chicken Caesar salad (skip the dressing), chicken sandwich (try to find one not breaded or fried) and eat only one side of the bun or bread. Some fast food restaurants have baked potatoes which you can get with chili or just eat the potato. My suggestion is to look up the menu of any restaurant prior to going out and make the choices that are healthy. This eliminates the temptation to buy a greasy burger and fries or other unhealthy options. By planning ahead, you will be able to continue eating healthy no matter where you are.

## MAKING HEALTHY EATING SIMPLE

Since 1994 I've been eating organic produce and eating very healthy. I have stayed the same weight, been in great health, and never had another polyp in my colon. By making quick healthy meals and learning how to stay on my meal plan no matter where I go, it is simple to eat healthy all of the time. It never takes me more than 10 minutes to make a great-tasting meal. I have enough food in my refrigerator and freezer to make a quick healthy meal.

Since everything I need is already cooked I can just reheat the food or eat it cold. A frying pan on the stovetop is the easiest way to heat up food. I personally don't like to microwave chicken or fish, but you can if you're in a hurry. Usually, there is time to reheat my food on the stovetop in a non-stick pan. Reheating vegetables in a non-stick pan over low heat takes only minutes whether they are already steamed or frozen. I use a steamer pot or put a steamer basket in any pan with a lid. Vegetables are cooked in a few minutes. (I never boil any vegetables in water because some of the nutrients are boiled out that way.) By putting a steamer basket in a pan, it keeps the vegetables out of the water. Steamer baskets are so small you can take them in your suitcase if you are going to be staying at a hotel that provides you with a stovetop.

Vegetables can also be cooked on a skewer with fish, chicken, tofu or just vegetables. My son cooks corn on the cob in the husk on his grill. He can cook chicken and corn at the same time. He is great at grilling and making fun meals for his family.

# Chapter 4: Tips for Losing Weight & Portion Control

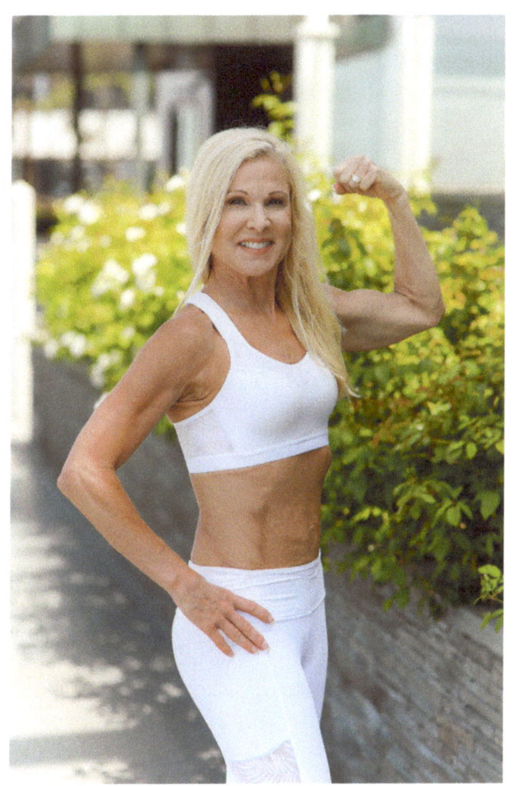

## EAT BEFORE AND AFTER EXERCISE

Eating before you exercise is very important, especially if you exercise in the morning. Your body has been resting and repairing during the night and it is important to hydrate and refuel in the morning. Drink a full glass of water with the juice of half a lemon when you wake up. Have a piece of Ezekiel toast with almond butter or Better Than Peanut Butter spread lightly with a small amount of organic fruit spread which is like jelly but it is made with just fruit. Another option is to put some low-fat cottage cheese on top of your toast which will give you energy for your workout. I keep some trail mix and some raw almonds in my gym bag. I always eat Ezekiel toast and veggie cheese, almond cheese or Better Than Peanut Butter with some fruit spread by Cascadian Farms, or another organic company, on my toast before I hit the gym.

My workout is usually one hour of cardiovascular exercise along with thirty or forty minutes of weight training and core exercises. I vary my workouts and if I feel tired or have an early appointment I cut down my cardiovascular exercise to thirty minutes.

After exercise it is important to have a healthy meal with a lean protein, complex carbohydrate, and small amount of fat. My breakfast is usually egg whites with vegetables and half a yam, thick or steel cut oatmeal with protein powder, cinnamon, a few slivered almonds, and fresh blueberries with Pure Stevia Leaf for sweetener. When I travel, I bring a baggie with cinnamon, stevia, slivered almonds, and dried dates along with a packet of protein to put on my oatmeal.

## CONTINUE HEALTHY EATING AND EXERCISE ALL YEAR LONG

When the weather gets cold, especially if you live somewhere where the weather is really too cold to go out for a walk, people tend to stay indoors. They do not do any exercise and they eat more which leads to weight gain. I call this putting on your winter coat.

Just because it is winter does not mean you should stop exercising and eating healthy. There are many options for eating healthy meals and for getting exercise even when it is cold or rainy outside.

Soups are excellent for lunch in cold weather and are very satisfying. Try making a vegetarian split pea soup or vegetable soup. Chicken soup is also a good choice. Dinner can be lean protein like chicken or fish, steamed vegetables, and brown rice or yams.

When the weather is nice and there are a lot of activities and outdoor events, it is much easier to exercise for some people. However, those dedicated to living a healthy life do not let a little cold weather stop them from exercising. Many people run in very low temperatures or find other activities they can do outside like snow skiing, snowboarding, and sledding. If you are sensitive to the cold and want to exercise indoors, there are many activities you can do at a gym. Jerry and I go to the gym all year long.

## AVOID MINDLESS EATING

When you are not eating healthy meals and snacks or waiting too long to eat, your body starts to crave something to get your blood sugar back up. Things that give a quick burst of energy may be very tempting if you don't understand how they spike your blood sugar and then drop it about an hour later. This can lead to mindless eating. Any time you eat something that is not good for you, consider that mindless eating.

When I first started writing this book, I considered the way people eat out of a large bag of chips or crackers. When the Lays Potato Chips commercial says *I bet you can't eat just one* they were right. People started eating them by the bagful. Many other unhealthy snacks were being eaten right out of the box or bag. The bags got larger and so did the people eating them.

By planning your meals and snacks and knowing portion sizes you can avoid mindless eating. Read the nutritional label and the ingredients. Ask yourself if you should be putting that into your body. For example, if a serving of cereal has more than 2-4 grams of sugar and is loaded with artificial colors, flavors, and preservatives, you should not be putting it into your body.

Choosing cereal that is nutrient dense and low in sugar with nothing artificial and no preservatives is simple and available at all grocery stores, not just organic food stores. Nature's Path has a great line of cereals. I love the Millet Rice Flakes that are gluten-free and very low in sugar. Another Nature's Path cereal that is gluten free is Purely O's which are very low in sugar. When I travel or go to an appointment I bring a baggie of cereal to eat if I get hungry. I always have food to eat when I leave the house. This keeps me satisfied until I have my next meal or snack. Bringing a lunch is always a good idea which helps avoid getting too hungry or eating fast food.

Teaching your children not to eat out of a large bag and to avoid junk foods is very important. Set a good example for your children so they grow up with good eating habits and don't have to struggle with their weight or a possible disease from overeating.

Forget about saying *save room for dessert*. If you are eating healthy foods and snacks you won't need desserts. This does not mean you cannot have dessert on a special occasion, but it does mean you stop eating sugary desserts that are loaded with sugar, fat, and extra calories. Desserts should be fruit salad with plain yogurt and Stevia or just a piece of fruit. Brown rice cakes or air popped or Skinny Pop popcorn is a good healthy treat. When you find healthy options to sugary desserts it is easy to stay healthy without feeling deprived.

Be sure your children are eating enough food to keep them from craving sugary desserts and chips. Many times the problem is they are not eating enough real food. When dinner is finished, wait for half of an hour for your brain to register whether you need more food. Making some frozen yogurt or ice cream with fresh fruit is a great treat. Buy an ice cream maker and teach your children how to make their own ice cream or frozen yogurt. It is simple to make and takes only about twenty minutes to make. That is less time than it takes to go out and buy ice cream.

I find that eating desserts during the day instead of at night helps keep the pounds off and helps my body relax at night. If you eat sugary snacks it is hard to keep from getting all wound up. Children get really wound up when they eat sugar. I hear parents say their kids are on a sugar high when they eat sugar and that is the truth. Many candy bars and protein or meal replacement bars have a lot of sugar and some have caffeine. By simply feeding them healthy snacks you avoid unnecessary problems that arise when kids are wound up on sugar. Find a recipe and replace all the unhealthy ingredients with healthy ones so you have your own bars to feed your kids. I created a recipe for my granddaughters for oat bars and we have been making them and eating them for years. They are a delicious family favorite.

Eating healthy foods will give you control over your health. Knowing when to eat and how much to eat is something that is controlled by your brain and hormones. If you are eating because you are bored, sad, lonely, or any other reason other than being hungry, that is mindless eating. When you feel stuffed, but don't know what you ate, this is also mindless eating. If you experience this it is important for you to recognize it and figure out why you are overeating. It may just be that you are eating too fast and your brain has not had the time to register that you are full. It takes about thirty minutes for your brain to register that full feeling. The habit of overeating or eating until you feel stuffed leads to obesity. By using portion control and eating slowly you can avoid overeating. Think about your food, and enjoy what you are eating. This will help eliminate mindless eating.

## QUICK TIPS FOR PORTION SIZES

The easiest way to exercise portion control is to make your lean protein the size of a deck of cards or the size of the palm of your hand. Carbohydrates that are starchy will be the size of your fist. This includes starchy vegetables like potatoes, winter squash, corn, yams, and grains like brown rice, quinoa, and all other grains. Eat as much non-starchy vegetables as you want. These include broccoli, cauliflower, celery, lettuce, spinach, cabbage, cucumber, zucchini, mushrooms, and more. All oils should be the size of the tip of your thumb and should be healthy oils such as extra virgin olive oil, and sunflower oil. Canola, sesame, walnut, grapeseed, and flaxseed oils are also great to use.

Use a 9-inch plate and divide it in half. Use one half for non-starchy vegetables. Divide the other half, using one quarter for your starchy vegetables or grains and the other quarter for your protein. Once you get used to seeing the size of your portions it will become easy to just look at what you are putting on your plate and know it is the right portion. (If you are eating cereal, use a measuring cup to see what a ½ cup or ¾ cup looks like in a bowl. It won't take long for you to be able to use the right amount without using a measuring cup.)

When you eat healthy, getting all the nutrients your body needs is very easy. Avocado has healthy fats, but also a lot of calories, so limit the amount you eat. Almonds are good for you, but they contain fat and a lot of calories, so limit the amount of any nuts you eat to a handful or eight nuts. Make sure you eat raw nuts and stick with the healthier nuts. Varieties such as almonds, walnuts, Brazil Nuts, and cashews are good choices. Eat a piece of fruit or something low in calories along with anything that is high in fat and calories which will help you limit the amount of the food that is higher in fat.

## AVOID FAD DIETS AND STARVATION DIETS

I have found that many people trying to lose weight use fasting or starvation as a way to cut calories. It is a common myth to think that not eating will create weight loss. It might work in the beginning because you lose water weight. When you fast or go long periods of time without eating, your body begins to store fat. This is your body's means of protection because it thinks you are starving, and it will slow down all processes to conserve energy. Eating less than 1,000 calories a day will slow down your metabolism causing your body to go into starvation mode burning muscle and storing fat. Repetitive fasting and long periods of time without food will put your body into fat-storing mode and ultimately fail to achieve the healthy weight loss results you hope for.

Carbohydrates are being eliminated by many fad diets, but they are essential for your body to function. Anyone who has stopped eating carbohydrates can tell you that it is very difficult because your body needs healthy carbohydrates. Healthy carbohydrates are vegetables, fruits, and 100% whole grains which have vitamins and fiber that the body needs. Beans and legumes have healthy carbohydrates, protein, and fiber. These are all nutrients that your body needs and uses.

What your body does not need is sugar, white flour, and white rice which break down very quickly and spike blood sugar. Because of their negative impact on blood sugar, the best thing to do is to avoid them.

Avoid these type of fad diets. By eating throughout the day, you will keep your metabolism running and continuously burning fat and calories. Add daily exercise to your healthy eating plan and you will have a lot of energy to take on everything you want to do.

## FOOD AND EXERCISE JOURNAL

One of the best ways to keep track of the foods you eat is to keep a food and exercise journal. There is something so powerful about writing things down on paper. It actually makes you think before you eat something because you know it has to go on your list. If you are gaining weight or just not getting to where you want to be, you can review your journal to see exactly what you are eating and what you might need to eliminate from your diet.

Writing down the type of daily exercise you do and its duration helps you understand how movement helps you maintain a healthy diet and lose weight faster. If you exercise daily but eat unhealthy foods, you won't reach your full potential. Focusing on diet only without adding exercise does the same thing.

When you eat a healthy diet and exercise you will improve your overall health, lose fat, have more energy, and sleep better at night. Start your food and exercise journal today and you will be motivated to continue eating healthy and exercising every day. You will enjoy the benefits of a healthy lifestyle!

## Choose Calories Wisely

Many people are confused about what calories are and why they are important. A calorie is simply a measure of energy. All foods and liquids, except water, have calories. Your body requires a certain number of calories to function and keep you alive. This is one of the reasons it is important not to restrict your calorie intake too much. As I said, your body will see this as a sign of starvation and start burning muscle and storing fat to protect itself. If you exercise, you will need to eat enough calories to provide additional energy for your exercise. The more you exercise the more you can eat without gaining weight as long as the foods you are eating are part of the healthy meal plan.

If you have a choice between a can of Coke and a bottle of orange juice (that have the same number of calories), is it okay to choose the Coke? The answer is NO. Orange juice provides vitamins, and many juices are fortified with calcium. Coke and other carbonated beverages are filled with sugar and high fructose corn syrup which add a lot of calories and promote tooth decay and weight gain. Coke and other carbonated beverages contain phosphorus which can decrease calcium levels. This, in turn, can weaken your bones.

The best choice when it comes to fruit versus juice is to always eat whole fruit. The fiber that is in fruit is very beneficial for your body and whole fruit has less sugar and fewer calories than juice.

Many juices have added sugar, high fructose corn syrup, and may have artificial ingredients. Read the label before you choose juice. Real juice and juice drinks are not the same. By reading the labels you will see the additional sugars and artificial flavorings and coloring in juice drinks. Drinking water and milk are better choices for kids and adults can have green tea which has many health benefits.

All calories are not created equal, and it is important to be informed about what you are putting into your body. The first three ingredients on the label are the ones that make up most of the product. Labels that list sugar or fat in the first few ingredients are usually higher in sugar than those placing sugar at the end of the list. If the label contains a long list of ingredients that you don't recognize, either look up the ingredients or just don't buy the product.

Birthday cake seems to be a big temptation for many people. I have not eaten birthday cake, or any cake for that matter, in over forty years. When Jerry and I got married, everyone at our wedding was wondering how we were going to do the part where we fed cake to one another. When he put the bite of cake in my mouth it was like a foreign object to me. My body is not used to eating things like cake so the one traditional bite was more than enough for me.

For the most part, if you do not have any food allergies or diabetes, you can have a piece of cake on rare or special occasions without it breaking your entire healthy eating plan. Avoid frosting because it is saturated fat and sugar with a lot of fat and calories. However, if cake (or whatever your weakness is) is a trigger food which makes you want to eat more of it, then it is best not to have any at all. Dessert can often be shared among three or four people if you are at a party or a dinner. Usually the portions are so large it is way too much for one person. I suggest each person get a bite or two, then it's, *forks down!* Everyone will be satisfied without loading up on calories, fat, and sugar for the day. If you are unable to eat just one bite take it completely out of your mind and don't eat any. After a while you won't miss it, especially when you see how good you look in a bathing suit when you stop eating sweets.

## THE TRUTH ABOUT TIME AND MONEY

If exercise and healthy eating are so good for us, why doesn't everyone do them on a daily basis? The answer to that question is usually because people don't think they have enough time or money.

However, exercising doesn't require buying a gym membership or expensive equipment. Daily exercise can be as simple as a brisk walk, hike, or run. Climb some stairs or find an exercise program on television, DVD, or online. Find something that motivates you. Choose dance music and dance around your living room. There are dance games that get you up and moving. Whatever gets you to take action and exercise daily will be of great benefit to your health.

Likewise, eating healthy does not require a lot of money if you look for organic produce on sale, go to a farmers market, or find out what stores have the best prices on organic foods. There are many grocery stores that carry organic produce, milk, eggs, and meats. By cutting out junk foods, sugary drinks, and things that are not good for your health (including tobacco and alcohol), you will save a lot of money that can be used for healthy foods.

## HOW TO EAT WHEN YOU TRAVEL

Travel has become very stressful, especially if you are flying. Tickets are very expensive and there are many additional fees once you get to the airport. There is a fee to check your bag and you are limited to what you can carry onto an airplane. If you buy food at the airport it is very expensive. When flights are delayed or canceled, it can cause a lot of stress and frustration.

Stress and costs can be greatly reduced by bringing your own food that is from this healthy eating plan. The night before a trip grill some chicken and make some sandwiches on Ezekiel bread to bring with you. Tuna comes in convenient pouches to travel with. I like to bring a Japanese or Garnet yam in my lunch bag to eat along with a chicken or tofu sandwich. When you are stuck on a plane you will be glad you have food to eat. Once you clear security, don't forget to buy bottled water. This will keep you hydrated throughout your travels. Having these healthy food choices with you while traveling keeps you from getting hungry and agitated. It will also keep you from eating whatever food you are able to find at the airport. This is a great way to make the flying experience more enjoyable, if you can afford to fly first class enjoy the larger seat, but still bring your own food. Food served on an airplane is not healthy. It has a lot of calories and has preservatives to keep it from going bad. Use the plate for your sandwich and the silverware to cut your yam. Enjoy the flying experience with my healthy foods to eat on the plane.

## Health Is Your #1 Priority

People can have many different reasons for wanting to lose weight. There are some who just simply want to look good in their swimsuits and shorts. Many people go to great lengths to lose weight like fasting, binge eating or other unhealthy ways to lose weight. Anorexia and bulimia have become serious problems for people who get into these unhealthy ways of losing weight and becoming thin. They begin to see themselves as fat no matter how much weight they lose. This is a very dangerous and serious problem that leads to psychological problems. By learning to eat healthy and keeping your body weight in a healthy range you can avoid getting into unhealthy ways of losing weight. When you learn to eat healthy you will lose weight, but not to the point of being stick thin. You want to look great and feel great while making health your number one priority. Don't lose sight of that for your family and yourself.

Heart disease and obesity are on the rise. Obesity is not only a problem for adults, but it has also become an epidemic among children. The problem is not that children have inherited the "fat genes" of their parents. They have adopted the bad eating habits of their parents. Set a good example for you family by always eating healthy foods and encourage them to eat healthy, too.

# CHAPTER 5: FOOD AND EXERCISE JOURNAL

My healthy eating plan includes keeping track of your daily food intake and exercise. This is a great way to keep you on target with your eating and fitness goals. When you write down everything you eat and drink as well as how you feel, it becomes very easy to establish what makes you feel great and what brings you down. There is something so powerful about writing things down on paper. It actually makes you think before you eat something because you know it has to go on your list of foods for the day. If you are gaining weight or just not getting to where you want to be, you can review your journal to see exactly what you are eating and what you might need to eliminate from your diet.

Writing down the type of daily exercise you do and its duration helps you understand how movement is part of maintaining a healthy diet and losing weight faster. If you exercise daily but eat unhealthy, you won't reach your full potential. Focusing on diet only without adding exercise will slow down the process of losing weight and you will not be getting all the healthy benefits of exercising. Another thing to keep in mind is that exercise is fun!

Through healthy eating and exercise along with keeping a daily journal, you will improve your overall healthy, lose fat, have more energy, and sleep better at night. Grab your journal and start writing. Enjoy the benefits of a healthy lifestyle!

There are many ways of tracking your progress. I suggest that you start by writing it down in the food and exercise journal page I have given you in this book. Make copies and put them in a binder. Do this in the beginning so you have a specific place to keep this information and you can review it without interruptions. When you use a tablet or computer it is easy to get distracted by calls, emails, and work. Once you are in the habit of eating healthy and exercising daily and have reached your fitness goals, you can continue tracking your progress in whatever format you want to. Be sure to back it up somewhere if you are going to use a tablet or computer so you don't lose it. Treat this as valuable information.

I even used this when I had surgery to look back to see what I had done years prior when I had a different surgery. Looking back at the daily progress I made walking during my recovery and what I ate as well as how I felt during my previous recovery was helpful. It was very motivating to see how much I walked every day and how I progressed day by day. Even though I was not doing the amount of exercise I was doing before surgery I was able to maintain my healthy weight by staying on my healthy eating plan and walking three times a day.

Anyone undergoing a surgery should consult their physician to see what the restrictions are post-surgery. Ask if you will be able to walk for exercise and how long you have to take off from your exercise program. Be very specific and do not do anything the doctor tells you to avoid. Not following orders can delay your recovery and keep you from exercise even longer.

If you are currently eating a diet that includes fast food, junk food, and sugary drinks, writing this down will help you eliminate all of them from your life. Being able to write down all the healthy foods and exercise you did for the day and how proud you feel of yourself raises your self-esteem.

I have been doing this for years even though I already eat healthy all of the time and exercise daily. I can look back over the years and see that I have been able to keep my weight stable and my eating healthy. The section for writing how you feel is important also. This is very helpful information when you are going through difficult times and for keeping track of recovery from an injury or surgery. This reference has helped me when dealing with doctors and even helped support my case after I was rear-ended by a car while sitting in traffic.

Using this food and exercise journal will help you stay motivated to eat healthy and exercise every day. If you have a cold it is okay to continue to exercise as long as it does not make you feel worse and you do not have anything that is contagious. If you have the flu you should stay home, drink plenty of fluids, and continue to eat healthy. Don't let feeling bad make you run to a tub of ice cream to make you feel better. Eat some homemade chicken soup which will always help you feel better.

When I make a pot of soup I put some in the freezer. There have only been a few times when I have been sick. I love my homemade chicken soup. I don't eat any other soup because I don't know what is in it and if it does have a label it usually has oil and things that don't need to be added to soup. I love to make soup during the winter months and put in a lot of vegetables to make a nutritious meal.

The journal also helps you track your weight and body fat. I recommend the Tanita Scale with body fat analysis. This scale reads not only weight, but percentage of body fat and the amount of water in your body. This is very helpful because, if you are dehydrated, it will let you know so you need to drink more water. Drinking water all day long, especially during exercise, will keep you hydrated.

I suggest weighing at least once a week. The best time of day to weigh is first thing in the morning. By weighing in at the same time each morning it will be easy to track your progress. Both the food and exercise journal and the scales are effective tools to help you stay on track.

When you write down what you eat, be sure to add *everything* you eat and drink. If you don't drink water all day long, start keeping track of how much water you drink until it becomes a habit. If you are already in the habit of drinking water throughout the day, especially during exercise and exertion, then you don't have to track your water consumption.

You *do* need to write down sodas, sweet tea, coffee, and any other drinks that have sugar, artificial sweeteners, artificial colors, or preservatives. The goal is to move away from all the artificial ingredients. Tracking the amount of caffeinated beverages you drink is very helpful because caffeine can affect your sleep pattern and has a diuretic effect which can make you dehydrated. Any type of caffeine supplements need to be written down as well. Log how you feel when you take them or if they kept you from falling asleep or if you wake often during the night. Some changes to how much caffeine and when you have it can help eliminate problems.

Alcohol is another thing that needs to go into the food journal. It has a lot of calories and it inhibits your ability to make good food choices. You may find that you eat more when you drink. One glass of wine has about 200 calories. That is the same as a boneless skinless chicken breast. This is how you will start to look at things which will encourage you to eat healthy and avoid alcohol.

As you change to my healthy eating plan and use this journal, you will note your progress, your weight loss, and how you feel along the way. This is all valuable information as you learn more about yourself. It is a very powerful way to cement healthy eating into your mind. It won't be long until making healthy food choices becomes a habit.

### HEART RATE MONITOR FOR EXERCISE

The body burns a greater amount of fat during lower intensity cardiovascular exercise over longer duration than it does during higher intensity. I have used a Polar heart rate monitor for you because it is a great way to track myself during my workouts.

I track my cardiovascular exercise such as using the treadmill or elliptical trainer by writing down the following information:

- Number of calories burned during exercise
- Exercise duration
- Average heart rate
- Time in fat-burning zone
- Percentage of fat calories burned

I usually do cardiovascular exercise before I lift weights to get my muscles warmed up. On the weekends I ride my spinning bike at home and then go to the gym. Some days I will just do cardiovascular exercise and ride my spinning bike. Cardiovascular exercise increases blood circulation throughout the body and also releases endorphins, the feel-good hormones which make you feel great. Some people like to do weightlifting first, and some like to do it after. Others like to do weights on one day and cardiovascular exercise the next day. As long as you do some form of warm-up before lifting weights, you can do whichever works best for you. Lifting weights and cardiovascular exercise will burn many calories while you are working out and building muscle will help your body burn more calories all day long. Both forms of exercise will greatly benefit your body and your overall health.

Writing down your daily food intake, exercise and weighing yourself once a week will give you all the information you need to figure out where you can improve. By going through your pages from the beginning to where you are in a few weeks or months later, your progress will amaze you and make you feel very proud of yourself.

## FOOD JOURNAL

Date:
Exercise Log:

| Food Diary<br>What I Ate | How I Felt |
|---|---|
| Breakfast | |
| Lunch | |
| Dinner | |
| Snack | |

Date:
Exercise Log:

| Food Diary<br>What I Ate | How I Felt |
|---|---|
| Breakfast | |
| Lunch | |
| Dinner | |
| Snack | |

# CHAPTER 6: FIBER, NUTS & OILS

## FIBER

Fiber can be either soluble or insoluble in nature and both types are necessary and beneficial for overall health and digestion. Foods that contain fiber are fruits, vegetables, 100% whole grains, beans, and legumes.

You can learn more about the benefits of fiber here: kidshealth.org/en/teens/fiber.html. It states that fiber can help lower blood cholesterol and prevent diabetes and heart disease. Eating carbohydrates that contain fiber helps slow the absorption of sugar and regulates insulin. Fiber also helps make you feel full which, in turn, helps reduce the amount of food you eat because you feel full longer.

Foods high in fiber are:

- Black beans
- Chick peas (garbanzo beans)
- Edamame (soy beans)
- Kidney beans
- Lentils
- Lima beans
- Navy beans
- Peas
- Refried beans
- Split peas
- Almonds
- Pistachios
- Coconut

- Walnuts
- Seeds
- Flax seeds/flax meal
- Quinoa
- All-Bran Cereal
- Barley Maize
- Brown rice
- Bulgur
- Oatmeal**
- Pearl Barley
- Popcorn
- 100% whole wheat bread
- 100% rye bread*
- Acorn squash
- Artichokes
- Brussels sprouts
- Carrots
- Kabocha squash
- Okra
- Parsnips***
- Potatoes (with peel)
- Sweet potatoes
- Vegetables
- Apples
- Avocados
- Bananas
- Blackberries
- Figs
- Oranges
- Pears

- Prunes
- Raisins
- Raspberries

* will be a smaller denser loaf usually found in the freezer section of health food stores
** thick oats, old-fashioned oats, Irish oats, steel-cut oats
*** can be added to soups and stews

Fiber is the part of a food that the body cannot digest or absorb. The website, livestrong.com [http://www.livestrong.com] (October 3, 2017), states that fiber can aid in decreasing the risk of heart disease and helps with digestion. It is very important to make fiber part of every meal in your healthy eating plan.

Soluble fiber dissolves in water and forms a gel-like material in the digestive tract that helps to lower cholesterol and maintain healthy blood sugar and cholesterol levels. Oats, barley, fruit, legumes (beans and peas), and psyllium contain soluble fiber. Insoluble fiber does not dissolve in water, so it adds bulk to the stool. Sources of insoluble fiber are wheat bran, whole grain breads and cereals, and many vegetables.

By eating a wide variety of vegetables and high fiber foods, you can be assured that you are getting a good amount of both types of fiber. Most plant-based foods contain both types of fiber. Fiber helps keep you regular and supplies a healthy balance to the gut. It assists in maintaining cardiovascular health and healthy blood sugar levels (that are already at a healthy level.) It also helps cholesterol levels that are already in the normal range to stay there.

By following my healthy eating plan and getting daily exercise, it is possible to regain healthy levels if you have high cholesterol. Eating healthy can help you avoid high blood sugar or blood sugar spikes. If you are already on medication for high cholesterol or high blood sugar, ask your doctor if you can lower your medication or even get off medication at some point by eating the way I suggest in my healthy eating plan. Be sure to mention that exercise is also a part of your healthy living plan to ensure there are no medical limitations your doctor wants you to follow.

Never try to stop medication on your own. If your doctor is not willing to help you meet your goals of reducing or eliminating the need for your medication, seek another opinion. Doctors should be happy that you are willing to follow a healthy eating and exercise plan. Doctors can help patients reduce and many times eliminate medications. If you are willing and able to reduce your cholesterol and lower blood sugar by making healthy lifestyle changes, it is possible to get off medications with the assistance of a medical professional.

My healthy eating plan is filled with fresh vegetables, fruits, beans, legumes, and 100% whole grains. This makes it easy to get the fiber needed to aid the body with elimination and to help protect it from disease.

## Flax Seed

Flax seed is a good source of dietary fiber along with omega-3 fatty acids. The fiber in flax seed is found primarily in the seed coat. The seeds can be ground in a coffee grinder or you can buy whole flax meal already ground. When you increase your fiber make sure to increase your water intake to help move the fiber through your system.

Add flax meal to protein shakes, smoothies, oatmeal, sauces, and baked goods. Flax seed meal helps you feel full. This can help you eat less. When it is ground, whole flax seed has 7.6 grams of both soluble and insoluble fiber. Flax seed also contains protein, polyunsaturated fatty acids, vitamin C, E, K, protein, potassium, calcium, and other beneficial minerals.

## Oils

There are many choices when it comes to deciding what oils to use for cooking. Some oils have become well known due to advertising. Some are just the latest fad. Canola oil is low in saturated fat and is good to use according to Sara Haas, RD, LDN, a chef in Chicago, and spokeswoman for the American Academy of Nutrition and Dietetics. She also recommends flaxseed oil, avocado oil, walnut oil, sesame oil, and grapeseed oil. (https://www.everydayhealth.com/news/ best-worst-oils-health/)

The USDA's database on food nutrition and safety declares, "It is best to follow the recommendations of the Dietary Guidelines for Americans and limit oils and saturated fats to less than 10 percent of your overall calories per day." (https://www.usda.gov/media/press-releases/2016/01/06/hhs-and-usda-release-new-dietary-guidelines-encourage-healthy).

Grapeseed oil has something that olive oil does not have, and that is linoleic acid levels. Research from Ohio State University indicates that high lipid content can lower your risk for heart disease and diabetes. Research suggests that taking as little as a teaspoon and a half of oil was all it took to increase lean body mass and reduce fat in the midsection.

Grapeseed oil is an excellent source of linoleic acid, constituting about 80 percent of its fatty acids. One tablespoon has 120 calories and 13.6 grams of fat (2.3 grams of saturated fat and 6.2 grams of monounsaturated fat, and 4.3 grams of polyunsaturated fat per the USDA. Grapeseed oil does well when cooking at high temperatures.

Use high quality oil such as olive oil or others on the list, but use sparingly. All you need is a teaspoonful; that's not much. Don't eat or fry your food. Deep frying adds a lot of fat and calories that you don't need in your diet or clogging up your arteries.

There is a variety of oils on the market, making it difficult to choose which one is best to use. Coconut oil is currently being marketed as the best oil to use for everything. Coconut oil is about 90% saturated fat. Butter contains up to 80% saturated fat which is less the amount in coconut oil. Too much saturated fat in the diet raises your "bad" LDL cholesterol. Another oil that is used in many products is palm oil. Palm oil is 50% saturated and has a fatty acid composition that makes it more flavorful than coconut oil or palm kernel oil. It is less saturated than butter and contains no trans-fat. The oil palm yields its extract from the flesh of the fruit (palm oil) and the other type is from the seed or kernel (palm kernel oil.)

Coconut oil has various applications and is popular because it is slow to oxidize and lasts up to six months without spoiling. One tablespoon of coconut oil has 117 calories, 14 grams of saturated fat, 0.2 grams of polyunsaturated fat and 0.8 of monounsaturated fat.

Palm oil is used in 50 % of products on supermarket shelves including food and nonfood products. Anything that has a coating such as a protein or meal replacement bar has palm or palm kernel oil in it. Palm oil has 120 calories per tablespoon, 14 grams of fat, 7grams of saturated fat, 1.3 grams of polyunsaturated fat, and 5 grams of monounsaturated fat.

Harvard Women's Health Watch from October, 2007, indicated that palm oil, made from the fruit of the oil palm tree, is one of the most widely produced edible fats in the world (https://www.health.harvard.edu/newsletter_article/By_the_way_doctor_Is_palm_oil_good_for_you). Tropical oils such as palm and coconut are plant-based. They do, however, have very different nutritional profiles than other plant-based fats do.

Saturated fat boosts "bad" cholesterol and triglycerides, both of which are risk factors for heart disease. When choosing which oil to use make sure to use one that is low in saturated fat or get your healthy fats from avocados, nuts, seeds, and fatty fish.

## NUTS

Nuts have many benefits when incorporated into a healthy diet. They contain both protein and healthy fats. You need to watch the amount you consume, however, because they are also high in fat and calories. Eat only raw nuts and limit the amount to a handful or eight to ten nuts. Don't eat roasted or salted nuts. The standard roasting processes significantly increase the trans-fat content and add more fat and calories.

# CHAPTER 7: MAKING A SHOPPING LIST & EASILY NAVIGATING THE GROCERY STORE

Are you frustrated when you go to the grocery store and end up buying things you do not want and do not need? This can happen very easily if you do not have a shopping list. One of the most helpful things to do before you go to the store is to create a shopping list. The list will have things you buy on a weekly basis and things that you only buy when needed. Perishable items such as fruits, vegetables, and dairy products are some of the things you will buy weekly. Proteins such as fish, seafood, chicken breast, ground turkey breast, and other proteins can be frozen and defrosted when needed. As you run out of things add them to your list. Visualize your grocery store when you make your list so you can write down items in the order they appear in the store. This keeps you from wandering around the store searching for what you want. It helps you stick to the healthy choices and saves you time in the process.

When you do not have a shopping list it is very easy to buy things that you do not need and things that are not good for you. If you bring your children to the store they will grab every sugary treat they see. Before you know it, you have a cart full of processed foods and sugary snacks. Making a list before you go to the store and sticking to it will eliminate the mindless shopping and extra expense of buying unnecessary products.

As I said before, start with a master grocery list that contains all the healthy foods. This should include lean proteins, complex carbohydrates, 100% whole grains, fruits, vegetables, and foods that contain healthy oils. Healthy options can be added to your list when you find new vegetables and fruits to try and new types of fish and vegetarian options. There is a lot of variety that can be added once you get into the habit of making healthy food choices.

A list of lean proteins such as fish, chicken breast, turkey breast, and ground turkey breast will be on your list. Beans and whole grain brown rice or quinoa, tempeh, or fermented tofu can turn any meal into a vegetarian option. Crab legs, lobster, shrimp, or tuna (fresh, frozen, or canned) are also good sources of protein. Eat a variety of protein and make some of your meals vegetarian by using brown rice or any 100% whole grain and beans. Quinoa is a grain that contains all nine essential amino acids, making it a complete protein. I recommend that you omit beef due to growth hormone, testosterone, and antibiotics given to cattle. Pork is advertised as the other white meat, but I recommend you avoid all types of pork. If you must eat beef use it occasionally and choose organic and the leanest cuts.

Fruits and vegetables are the main part of my healthy eating plan. They are full of nutrients, phytochemicals, and fiber, among other things. There are starchy and non-starchy vegetables. Starchy vegetables are winter squash, potatoes, yams, Japanese yams, and corn along with some other vegetables. Non-starchy vegetables such as broccoli, cauliflower, asparagus, celery, lettuce, spinach and other leafy greens, and cabbage are nutrient dense and have very few calories. Eat as many of these as you wish as long as you don't add any butter or oil. (Fat has almost twice the calories of complex carbohydrates. By omitting oils and butter you are greatly reducing the calories in your meal.)

Grains are complex carbohydrates that are starchy. Using 100% whole grains reduces the starch and increases the fiber and nutrients. Use 100% whole grains such as brown rice, quinoa, oatmeal, rye, and others. Breads are also included in this list. It is best to find flourless, 100% whole grain bread that you like. The two that I find the healthiest are Ezekiel bread and tortilla shells or Alvarado Street breads and tortilla shells.

Fats and oils are also on the list, as long as they are healthy options. Some choices of oils are extra virgin olive, canola, flaxseed, avocado, walnut, sesame, or grapeseed oil. All of your fat requirements can come from foods such as walnuts, almonds, avocados, salmon, and other fatty fish. Most people get plenty of fat in their diet. Make sure the fat you are getting from your diet is healthy fat.

Now you know what healthy foods to include on your shopping list. Next I will teach you how to navigate the grocery store and how to avoid buying foods that are not good for you.

## Don't Shop Hungry

Never shop when you are hungry. This is something that will help you stick to your list and make healthy food choices. Everyone knows what happens when you shop when you are hungry. You end up buying everything that looks good and will give you a quick pick-me-up. This is always in the form of sugary snacks or processed foods that are easy to make and eat quickly. By eating something before you go shopping you can avoid the mindless shopping that happens when you are hungry. This will also help you say no to the free samples you find in the store. When you aren't starving you aren't tempted to buy or eat things that are not good for you and shopping is much easier!

## Ignore Television Commercials

Foods and snacks that are advertised on television are mostly sugary cereals and snack foods that should be avoided, too. Advertisers are very skillful at targeting people who are home during the day and children. They create commercials that stick in your head and your children do not forget. Children are heavily marketed to by advertisers pushing their surgery cereals and snacks. Limit television watching for you and your children to avoid being a target to advertisement of sugary products.

## Shop the Perimeter Aisles

Yes, for the most part, the healthy foods are located on the perimeter of the store. This includes the weekly basics such as fruits, vegetables, dairy products, lean proteins, and bulk beans, split peas, brown rice, quinoa and other 100% whole grains. Ezekiel and Alvarado Street breads and tortillas are found in the frozen section.

Buy your big products such as laundry soap, bath soap, paper towels, toilet paper, and bathroom cleaners at the big warehouse stores to save money by buying in bulk. This also keeps you out of the center aisles of the regular stores where the temptations of processed foods, candy, and chips are located. Until you are in the habit of not buying these things avoid the aisles that contain them.

When my husband, Jerry, and I go to Costco, for example, we are on a mission. We bring a list and we stick to it! The first place we go to is the fish department, then around to the paper products. From there we head to the canned tuna, then to the laundry soap before heading right to the checkout registers. Costco is where we buy our big items that go in the pantry and freezer and we complete that task in a matter of minutes. Everything else we buy during the week comes from an organic food store, farmers market, or regular store that carries organic products.

## Bring Your Shopping List to the Store

Your shopping list can be on a piece of paper or written on your phone as long as it is with you when you go to the store. Check to make sure you have everything that you need on your list before you leave the house. This will keep you on track when you start shopping.

If you forget your list take a few minutes to write another one that includes everything that you remember writing down. When you write things down it anchors them in your mind. You can visualize what you wrote down and make a new list.

There have been times when I have forgotten my list, but I always have a pad of paper in the car to write things down. When this happens, I sit in the car and write down everything I can remember and think of what ingredients I need to make several meals for the week.

When you get into the habit of buying healthy foods all the time it will be easy to remember what you need. Even if you do forget something, you will have many alternatives to use either at home or on your new list. When you write the list think of how many different meals you can make with each type of protein. There are many options if you forget to buy one or two things because you have already figured out a number of meals instead of just thinking of one or two meals at a time.

If you have children, teach them how to shop and how to follow a list. Go over the list with them and make it a game to find items in the order they appear in the store. If you don't do this, you may find yourself chasing kids down the sugary snack aisle. Avoid the melt down at the check stand. Teach your kids how to be healthy food finders and they will enjoy helping.

I have young granddaughters and they love to go to the farmers market and grocery shopping. I teach them to make healthy food choices and let them put fruits and vegetables in the bag for me. I don't let them run through the store grabbing whatever they want. I know they love fruits, berries, tofu, yams, and broccoli. They love Amy's Bean & Rice Burritos, which are in the frozen section. They are also fans of Amy's or Muir Glen organic salsa. They enjoy helping me make the shopping choices as we go through the healthy aisles of the store. I go over the shopping list with them before we go into the store. They also go through the coupons to see if there is a sale on things we usually buy. We do it together and make it fun.

Try this with your children. It not only makes the shopping experience less hectic for you, but also saves you a lot of time and money. And what better way to start teaching them how to make healthy food choices?

## Educational Shows about Food Choices

The fast food industry has created the fast food mentality where the faster you can get and eat the food, the better it is for everyone. People have been convinced that getting quick meals that are already prepared is easy and convenient. Kids are convinced that getting a free toy makes fast food the best choice.

Last year McDonald's sold billions of Big Macs according to their latest commercial celebrating the launch of the Big Mac. When given a choice of where to eat, many kids will say McDonald's because they want a Happy Meal. This is a precooked hamburger that comes with French fries and a free toy. I would like to point out that the toy is not free because you have to buy the meal to get the toy and the meal is not something to be very happy about when you consider how many calories, grams of fat, and the amount of sodium in the meal. (A happy meal weighs in at 365 calories, 14 grams of fat, 560 mg sodium, 48 grams of carbohydrates, 14 grams of protein, and 10 grams of glucose.)

Knowing what you are eating and the nutritional values, which must be presented to you if you request them, is extremely important. You can also look up this information on the computer. *Fast Food Nation* and *Super-Size Me* are shows that give you an idea of what is happening in America due to fast foods, processed foods, junk foods, and sodas. HBO had a documentary called *Weight of the Nation* which focuses on the obesity epidemic in America.

Another HBO documentary series, *Weight of the Nation Kids*, focuses on obesity in children and how it affects their health, social life, and ability to function as a kid. Obesity affects one in three children. Children are suffering with their weight along with high blood pressure, type-2diabetes, high cholesterol, heart disease and more. These are diseases that were only seen in adults in the past. Children are worried about their own weight as well as the weight and health of their parents and family members.

## What Are the Best Vegetables to Buy?

To ensure getting a healthy amount of nutrients and fiber, buy a variety of vegetables in a wide array of colors. Non-starchy vegetables are very low in calories. As long as you eat them plain, you may eat as many as you want. I recommend that you eat cruciferous vegetables because of their cancer-fighting nutrients–broccoli, cauliflower, cabbage, Brussels sprouts, to name a few.

Green leafy vegetables like spinach, bok choy, kale, and collard greens are excellent choices. Lettuces are also good, such as romaine and butter lettuce. Artichokes, asparagus, and green beans help round out the group.

Starchy vegetables such as corn, carrots, green peas, plantains, potatoes, sweet potatoes, and winter squash (acorn, kabocha, and butternut) are great choices. These vegetables should be a part of your diet because they are loaded with fiber, vitamins, and nutrients.

When looking for vegetables, don't be afraid to try new things. Bell peppers are red, green, and yellow. Onions that are brown, white, red or green onions can be used to add flavor. They add a lot of color and flavor to your vegetable dishes. Some vegetables that you might not like to eat by themselves might taste great in a stew or mixed with other vegetables. Try what I call a *stir-unfry* (using no oil).

## What Are the Best Fruits to Buy?

Fruit is a great choice to eat all year long, and it is one that most children love. Eating fruit is a much better choice than eating sugary treats or even drinking fruit juice. When you eat the whole fruit, you get all the nutrients, phytochemicals, and fiber.

There are a few things to know about buying fruits (and some vegetables) before you go to the store or farmers market. Keep these simple rules in mind when you shop:

1. Fruits that have a hard-outer layer (i.e., melons) can be bought either locally grown or non-organic.
2. The *Dirty Dozen* should be bought organic if at all possible.

The *Dirty Dozen* include the following produce items:

- Strawberries
- Spinach
- Nectarines
- Apples
- Grapes
- Peaches
- Cherries
- Pears
- Tomatoes
- Celery
- Potatoes
- Sweet bell peppers

Try to find a farmers market or store that carries a variety of fresh fruits and vegetables that are not in cold storage bins. Fruits from the farmers market are usually ripe, so buy only what you will use in a week or can store in the refrigerator. Berries can be frozen and used for smoothies or frozen yogurt recipes. Frozen bananas are great for smoothies, frozen yogurt, or to eat like a Popsicle.

Fruits that are higher in sugar content such as bananas and watermelon may cause a spike in blood sugar. Eat them with other fruits to limit the amount you consume or have some protein like Greek yogurt or some healthy fat like almonds or cashews. Low-fat cottage cheese is good to eat with fruit, too.

Fruit can be eaten as a snack by itself or with a few nuts or low-fat cottage cheese. If you are trying to lose weight or find that you feel hungry an hour after eating fruit, eat some protein with it. Try chopped apples in low-fat cottage cheese which is really good for a quick snack.

Make a fruit salad by cutting up a few different kinds of fruit. It will stay fresh in the refrigerator if you plan on eating it the same day. If you use fruits like bananas and pears which turn brown within a day or two, store them in separate containers or just cut what you will eat in one sitting. Tupperware or glass storage containers with an airtight lid are good for storing leftover fruit. Apples, oranges, and hard fruits are best left on the countertop or fruit bowl. Remember that, after you cut into fruit, it must be refrigerated.

## What Type of Tofu Should I Buy?

Tofu comes in many different types determined by the amount of soy protein each contains. The consistency choices are *silken*, *soft*, *firm*, and *extra firm*. Each one is better-suited to some cooking styles and recipes than others. The best way to learn how to use them is to follow recipe recommendations, where available, and by simply trying them out to see what tastes right for you.

Silken tofu can be used to make things taste creamy, such as smoothies, salad dressing, or sauces. It can be used instead of eggs in recipes, and it can be used instead of meat in sauces and stir-fry. I use extra firm tofu when I make a meatless vegetable dish. Fermented tofu is also called fermented bean curd. It is used in Chinese cuisine and is made with soybeans, salt, rice wine, and either sesame oil or vinegar. Plain tofu has no flavor, so whatever type of sauce, vinegar, Bragg's Liquid Amino Acids, Tamari soy sauce or light soy sauce, or whatever flavoring you use is what the tofu will taste like.

There are some types of tofu that come already flavored. These can be sliced and put on sandwiches or eaten right out of the package. My granddaughters love the teriyaki tofu. I always bring it when I visit them or when we take a trip together. It is very easy to travel with and can stay out of the refrigerator longer than chicken or other perishable meats.

## What about Organic or Grass-fed Beef?

You will find some helpful information on this subject by checking out the following link:

http://nationalaglawcenter.org/usda-ams-pulls-standard-grass-fed-naturally-raised-meat. There has been action taken over the last few years concerning "grass-fed" beef. The above website will give you the Agricultural Marketing Service (AMS) standings on the USDA position on the marketing and labeling of grass-fed and naturally raised meats. There is no longer any governing body that regulates the claims for grass fed or the labeling of the products. Free range is another term used in marketing and labeling. This does not mean the product is organic.

## Should I Buy Organic?

The answer can be found by visiting this website: https://www.usda.gov/media/blog /2012/03/22/organic-101-what-usda-organic-label-means. In order for anything to be Certified Organic it has to follow the standards set by the USDA.

I personally buy organic dairy products like eggs, low-fat cottage cheese, Greek yogurt, milk, organic chicken, grains, and produce. I have been on 100% organic foods since my diagnosis of colon cancer in 1994. Since 1994 I have had no recurrence of cancer or even a polyp in my colon. My overall health is great and I feel great and I don't worry about unhealthy chemicals in the food I eat.

Buying organic produce, especially the ones that contain the most pesticides and herbicides. Buy dairy products and meat products that are organic. Cut out the sodas and sugary juice drinks and buy bottled water or install a water filter at home which will save you a lot of money. There is always a way to afford organic products if you cut out the things you don't need and those that are unhealthy,

## Best Bread to Eat

Eating the right type of bread is very important due to the fact that the majority of breads are made with mostly white flour along with artificial ingredients and preservatives.

The only bread I buy is Ezekiel sesame, Ezekiel raisin, and Alvarado Street breads. Both brands are Certified Organic and flourless. I love Alvarado Street California-style bread. Food for Life Ezekiel Breads are Certified Organic, made with sprouted grains, beans, and lentils, and all the ingredients from the Bible found in Ezekiel 4:9. They taste great and are loaded with nutrients.

Both brands also have tortilla shells that are nutrient dense and can be found in the frozen section of the store. I mostly eat Ezekiel bread and tortillas. Food for Life is the brand that makes Ezekiel bread and gluten-free breads. I love the Raisin Pecan bread. It tastes great with almond cheese or Marmalade fruit spread which is made from just the fruit. If you are used to eating white flour breads and tortillas, Alvarado Street bread and tortillas are softer and less dense than Ezekiel breads. I encourage you to try both and have your family eat them also. They are very crunchy when toasted and are very satisfying. Neither brand has any preservatives in them, only healthy ingredients. These breads are denser and not spongy like regular breads which have very little whole grain if any at all, and also have preservatives and artificial ingredients along with sugar and other ingredients that do not need to be in bread.

## Running Late or Don't Have Much Time?

There are many healthy choices at the store that you can buy to make a quick meal. Most stores have a cold section with prepared salads. Buy a salad with chicken and leave off the salad dressing which adds a significant amount of calories. They have Amy's Bean & Rice Burritos which are organic and have a whole-wheat tortilla. Try brown rice bowls. There are many healthy alternatives to grabbing a burger and fries. Many stores have a microwave that you can use to heat your food in.

Many times, I had to improvise when I left my lunch at home or my morning became afternoon before I knew it. That is when I find some Ezekiel Sesame bread, seasoned tofu and ask the deli in the store for some mustard and a piece of lettuce. I make my own sandwich right there in the store. This is really easy if they have a section with tables where people can sit and eat. I bought an Amy's Bean and Rice Burrito and asked if they would microwave it at the deli when they did not have a microwave in their lunch area. Premade salads or a salad bar has a lot of options for a quick lunch and I love the rice paper rolls or vegetable rolls that are in the sushi section of the store. Vegetable rolls are great with some sashimi, raw sushi grade fish, or ask the sushi chef to make a vegetable roll with tuna in it. There are so many healthy options which do not involve a burger and fries.

If you are craving a burger, look for a healthier option such as veggie burger or turkey burger. You can make them at home and have them in the refrigerator or freezer. For frozen patties wrap them in a wet paper towel and cook for a few seconds in a microwave or heat on low in a frying pan on the stovetop. Use Ezekiel bread instead of a bun which cuts a lot of calories out of the meal also. Toast your bread and eat your sandwich open faced using one piece of bread instead of two and use a leaf of lettuce for the top.

Organic egg whites bought in a carton can be turned into a quick meal. Microwave them for 2-3 minutes for scrambled eggs. Add some Yukon Gold potatoes and frozen vegetables to make a whole meal low in calories and rich in nutrients.

I am an expert at quick meals. Jerry and I had to move twice when his duty station changed. Both times we only had 30 days. We did not have time to find a house to rent, so we moved into a hotel for a month. I cooked all our meals in the microwave. We had a tiny refrigerator and a cooler, so we had to go to the store and buy enough for a few days at a time.

In central Texas in 2003, there were not a lot of choices when it came to organic and vegetarian cuisine. I stayed a vegetarian ten years, but once we left California it was hard to find tofu and other foods I loved to eat. I started eating fish, eggs, and yogurt to get my protein. Luckily, there was the original Whole Foods Market in Austin which was an hour away. My aunt and uncle just moved there, so I could go visit them and then go grocery shopping at Whole Foods.

It is possible to eat healthy wherever you are if you look for healthy foods. Make fruits and vegetables the main part of your meals, then add a starch (yams, squash, quinoa, brown rice) and a lean protein. That is all there is to it.

## Tracy's Master Shopping List

Use my master shopping list and see how easy it is to eat healthy with what you buy at the store. It is so easy and inexpensive; you will wonder why you didn't think of this yourself. It does not take any more effort to eat healthy and live a healthy lifestyle. There are so many benefits to doing so. It won't take you long to see changes in yourself and in your family. It is a great feeling to know that you have made positive changes in your life. Here's my list:

- Spinach
- Romaine lettuce
- Tomatoes
- Avocados
- Carrots
- Celery
- Beets
- Parsley
- Asparagus
- Broccoli
- Cauliflower
- Cucumber
- Zucchini
- Japanese yams
- Jewel yams
- Yukon gold potatoes
- Acorn squash
- Kabocha squash
- Delicata squash
- Bananas
- Apples
- Oranges
- Strawberries
- Raspberries
- Blackberries
- Blueberries
- Papaya
- Mango

- Teriyaki tofu
- Firm organic tofu
- Almond, soy veggie or heart-smart cheese
- Dried navy beans
- Dried pinto beans
- Lentils
- Split peas
- Lima beans
- 100% whole grain pasta
- Organic chunky tomato sauce
- Organic stewed tomatoes
- Almond butter
- Better Than Peanut Butter
- Simple Fruit
- Salmon
- Sea bass
- Shrimp
- Organic ground turkey breast
- Organic chicken, boneless & skinless
- Nature's Path gluten-free Millet Rice Flakes
- Nature's Path Purely O's
- Red's Oatmeal
- Red's gluten-free oat flour
- Pure Stevia Leaf
- Xylitol
- Spring water, large jugs
- Organic eggs
- Low-fat milk
- Unsweetened almond milk
- Organic Greek yogurt, low-fat

- Organic low-fat cottage cheese
- Frozen Amy's bean & rice burritos
- Frozen mixed vegetables
- Frozen stir-fry vegetables
- Frozen California-style vegetables
- Ezekiel sesame bread
- Ezekiel raisin bread
- Alvarado Street California-style bread
- Ezekiel or Alvarado Street tortillas, large & small
- Amy's or Muir Glen medium salsa
- Agave ketchup
- Bearitos low-fat vegetarian refried beans
- Bearitos low-fat vegetarian refried black beans
- Kidney beans
- Garbanzo beans & artichoke hearts
- Tuna packed in water
- Relish (unsweetened)
- Organic brown rice cakes, lightly salted
- Deli turkey breast, 1 pound, nitrate/antibiotic/hormone-free, oven roasted, sliced thick

The protein that I am going to use for the next three days is put into the refrigerator. Canned and dried beans go into the pantry along with the pasta and canned tomatoes. Tortillas and bread go into the freezer to keep them fresh for as long as possible. I thaw them as I need them. Berries get stored in Tupperware on top of a paper towel. This helps them stay fresher longer. Remember to rinse them when ready to eat, not before storing. There is a type of Tupperware with a strainer at the bottom which is great for any type of melon and pineapple. It keeps them fresh longer. Potatoes go in the pantry along with squash and yams or on the counter next to the fruit bowl. All whole fruit goes into the fruit bowl or on the countertop. When they get really ripe, I put them into the refrigerator. Any fruit or berries that are almost overripe, I put into the freezer to use in smoothies and frozen yogurts.

I can make a large variety of meals with what I have on this list, including vegetarian meals. And I have food in the freezer and in the pantry. I always have enough food in the house to make a healthy meal so I never need to run out to the store at the last minute. And I never go out for fast food. I can make a quick healthy meal at home for a fraction of the cost of fast food, and I don't have to drive anywhere.

# Chapter 8: Reading Labels, Understanding Nutritional Information & What to Avoid

Reading food labels can be very difficult unless you know what to look for. It has become more complicated as the Food and Drug Administration (FDA) allows manufacturers to label products with wording that sounds confusing. As a basic rule of thumb, if the name of an ingredient is very long and complicated, it is probably something you should not buy. There are a lot of artificial ingredients, preservatives, and chemical additives added to foods to prolong their shelf life. These chemicals have been approved by the FDA, but that does not mean they are good for you. Avoid these chemicals and high fructose corn syrup, monosodium glutamate, trans-fats, and foods that are high in sugar and fats.

Likewise, if you eat something that doesn't taste like it only has 1 gram of sugar or doesn't taste like it is low in fat, be sure to read the label and check out the ingredients. It seems that manufacturers are finding new ways of labeling products that may be misleading for some people. There is a difference between sugar-free and "no sugar added." Sugar-free products usually have artificial sweeteners and "no sugar added" is not sugar-free. It just means that additional sugar has been added to the amount of sugar already in the product. A label can say zero grams of sugar if it has 0.5 grams or less of sugar per serving. (The same is true for products labeled fat-free. If there is 0.5 grams of fat or less per serving it can be labeled zero fat on the package.)

Make sure to look at the serving size and see how much sugar or fat there is per serving size. I was looking at a product that claimed it was a low-fat and high-protein ice cream. It was the smallest container on the shelf and it had 120 calories per serving. Many people would assume that a serving would be the whole little container. When I checked the serving size it said 3.5 per container. Do your math and figure out the total calories per container which is 120 X 3.5 = 420 calories in the small container. In a half cup there is 120 calories, 1.5 grams of fat, 20 milligrams of cholesterol, 19 grams of carbohydrate, 3 grams of fiber 9 grams of sugar, 7 grams of sugar alcohol. Xylitol is an example of a sugar alcohol that is a naturally occurring sugar alcohol that comes from fruits and vegetables. It is widely used as a sugar substitute and has only a third the calories of regular sugar. Xylitol is used in gums, mints, sugar-free candy, and more. As you read the labels you will see that many manufacturers use a combination of sugar and sugar alcohol in products to cut down the calories and the amount of sugar. Xylitol does not harm your teeth the way sugar does.

I bought some Purc Stevia Leaf, which is what I use on oatmeal and in baking. When I opened the container, I noticed that the product looked like sugar granules instead of a fine powder, which is what it usually looked like. When I read the label, the first ingredient in the list was maltodextrin, then stevia. There was more maltodextrin in it than there was stevia (the amount of the ingredient is indicated by its order in the label's list).

Maltodextrin is a polysaccharide that is used as a food additive. It is produced from starch by partial hydrolysis and is usually found as a white, hygroscopic, spray-dried powder. It is easily digestible, being absorbed as rapidly as glucose, and may be either moderately sweet or almost flavorless, depending on its use.

Maltodextrin is a product found in many packaged products such as certain brands of yogurt, sauces, and salad dressings. It lacks nutritional value and there are healthier options. It is used as a thickener, filler, or preservative in many processed foods.

Maltodextrin can cause spikes in blood sugar, even higher than table sugar. The side effects are like most food additives which include allergic reactions, unexplained weight gain, bloating, and flatulence. Specific allergic reactions could be rash, asthma, itching, and difficulty breathing.

Sugars can be identified on packaging labels because they usually end is -*ose* (fructose, glucose, lactose, etc). Maltodextrin is the exception to the rule.

Even if you look for the amount of sugar per serving, it can still be misleading because all the types of sweeteners may not be included in that amount of sugar. The amount of table sugar is counted in the amount of sugar per serving, but that may not be the total amount of sugar in the product. This is a really great reason why eating foods in their natural state is the best way to know what you are eating.

You can take any food or recipe and turn it into something healthier. By using real ingredients, you can create wonderful low-fat, low-sugar, or no-sugar-added versions. That does not mean that you use artificial sweeteners like Splenda. Choose stevia which has no calories and is good for you.

Some people try stevia once and decide they don't like it. If you experience this, use less until you get used to the taste. Using stevia in place of sugar really cuts down on the calories you consume. It's a great choice for diabetics because it doesn't spike blood sugar levels like sugar does. Stevia also does not promote tooth decay like sugar does.

You can also use xylitol. It does not promote tooth decay. You will see it in the ingredients of many health foods, mints, and gum. It is not harmful to body. Xylitol is not calorie-free, but it has 1/3 fewer calories than sugar which makes it a great option alongside stevia.

Both these healthier sweeteners can be purchased in serving-sized packets. Carry them with you so you have them available all through your day. They are a great help if you are out somewhere and want to sweeten a beverage without using sugar or an artificial sweetener. I advise you to carefully read the labels on everything until you know what is in the foods and products you consume.

## MORE REASONS TO EAT ORGANIC

By eating an all-organic diet it is easier to make sure you stay away from additives, artificial colors, and artificial flavorings. Organic crops are grown with fewer pesticides and harmful fertilizers. Organic livestock and poultry are raised without the use of dangerous hormones and synthetic chemicals. Organic rules also apply to products that are made from berries or grains. If baby food or jam is labeled organic, there are many chemicals that are not allowed in these products.

Organic is only strictly regulated by the National Organic Program (NOP) when it is produce or agriculture. Organic products like soaps or lotions that are labeled "organic" are not regulated in the same way. There are two different certifications that mean two different things. If the product has the United States Department of Agriculture (USDA) seal of "Certified Organic," it has been certified to contain 95% or more organic ingredients. Compare that to a product whose label states "made with organic ingredients." These products can have 70% of those ingredients certified as organic (See https://www.usda.gov/media/blog/2016/07/22/understanding-usda-organic-label).

When you go to a farmers market look for the "Certified Organic" sign which means they have to follow the government standards. If you see just the word certified, it is not Certified Organic.

Many products also say "all natural." That really does not mean anything because there are no regulations governing the use of this term on the label.

Some health food stores claim that they do not have any artificial colors or flavors. And many stores have come out with their own line of organic products. When you shop, look for the Certified Organic seal which will help ensure you are really getting certified organic produce and along with meats and poultry that are raised under the rules which allow them to carry that seal.

Knowing what you put into your body is key to maintaining your health, so don't be fooled by labels that have no governing body controlling and monitoring them. When buying foods other than the ones I mention or anything that you are not sure about make sure to read the label.

## PROTEIN BARS

Protein bars and meal replacement bars are basically just candy bars in most cases. If you look at the nutritional value of the bars in the store, you will see how much sugar, salt, fat, and calories are in them. They are also likely to make you crave sugar because they can raise your blood sugar and then drop it again. If you avoid sugar, you will not experience the crash you get about an hour later or the craving for more.

Fig bars were thought to be healthy but if you read the label you will see how much sugar and artificial ingredients are in them. I was given one on an airplane and I read the label. This fig bar had 220 calories with 40 of those coming from fat. It contains 5 grams of fat, 70 mg of sodium, 40 grams of carbohydrates, 4 grams of fiber, 20 grams of sugar, and 4 grams of protein... and it is loaded with bad ingredients and trans-fats.

A Kashi bar called Honey, Almond, & Flax sounds like it would be healthy. Yet it has 140 calories with 45 of them coming from fat, 1.4 grams polyunsaturated fat, 2.5 grams monounsaturated fat, 105 mg of sodium, 19 grams of carbohydrates, 4 grams of fiber, (1-gram soluble fiber, 3 grams insoluble), 5 grams of sugar, and 7 grams of protein.

A Luna bar (without chocolate coating on the bottom) has 170 calories, with 40 coming from fat. They contain 4.5 grams' total fat, 180 mg of sodium, 26 grams of carbohydrates, 3 grams of fiber, 11 grams of sugar, 12 grams of other carbohydrates, and 9 grams of protein. The ingredients in this bar are healthier than most bars.

A Lara bar is made of just fruit and nuts and has 230 calories, 110 from fat. It has 1.5 grams of saturated fat, 0 grams of trans-fat, 2.5 grams of polyunsaturated fat, 8 grams of monounsaturated fat, 5 mg of sodium, 23 grams of carbohydrates, 3 grams of fiber, 18 grams of sugar, and 6 grams of protein. This is the cashew cookie flavor; values may vary depending on the flavor.

The bottom line is that you need to read the ingredients and check the amount of fat, calories, sugar, and protein to make an informed decision on whether you want to eat a bar or eat some fruit, plain Greek yogurt with fresh berries and stevia or just have a small meal like a chicken breast with broccoli.

## SOY...TO EAT OR NOT TO EAT

Whether or not you eat soy is up to you. If you do decide to eat it, make sure it is fermented and of high quality. Many products have soy in them, but this is not the same as tempeh or fermented tofu. Not all soy is the same.

It is best to use soy when it is fermented and consumed in moderation. Eating good quality soy can help to fight against some types of cancer and may help survivors of prostate cancer. Survivors eating a high-fiber diet can help lower their risks of colon cancer.

Soy foods such as edamame and tempeh have plenty of roughage. According to alive.com, fermented soy has friendly bacteria or probiotics that help the gut and digestive flora.

If you have severe allergies or any other concerns about eating soy, consult your doctor before adding it to your diet. Fermented soy can increase vitamins and minerals. Some of the yeast used in the fermentation process adds large quantities of thiamin, nicotinic acid, and biotin which also help make fermented soy the healthiest choice.

# CHAPTER 9: TEACHING YOUR CHILDREN HOW TO EAT HEALTHY

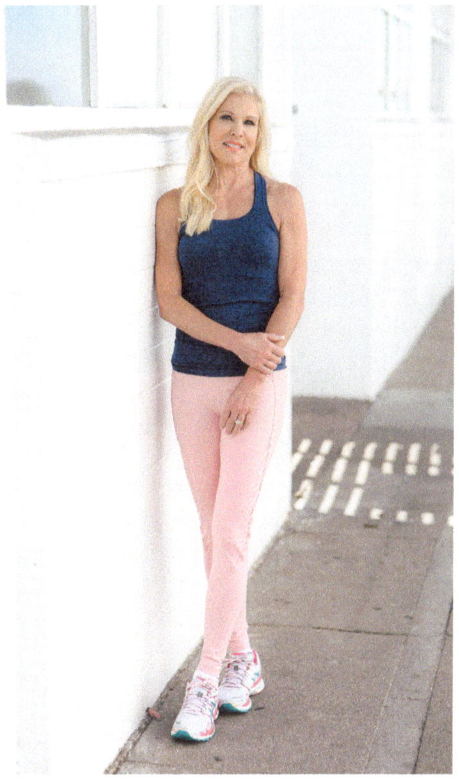

Teaching your children and grandchildren how to eat healthy is essential to their health and well-being. They are little sponges thirsty for knowledge. They will do whatever they are told, and they learn by example. Set a great example for your children by preparing and eating healthy at every meal. If kids are brought up eating healthy, they will know what to eat when they are away from home. Eating healthy foods creates a lasting impact on the entire family that will carry them throughout their lives.

Jamie Oliver's *Food Revolution* is one of the greatest examples of the problem with the American diet and school lunches. Jamie is a professional chef from England who created a documentary called *Food Revolution*. In it, he visited various schools in the United States to see why the lunches were so unhealthy. He talked with the children to find out what they thought was healthy and to learn what they were being served for lunch in the cafeteria. (https://abc.go .com/shows/jamie-olivers-food-revolution)

The children did not like the lunches, and they even had concerns about their health and the health of their family members. Many of the children were obese or had parents or family members who were obese, had type-2 diabetes, heart disease, high blood pressure, or high cholesterol. Some of the children were already suffering from the same diseases as the adults.

One in three children in the United States is or will become obese, and the numbers are rising. Some of the children in this documentary were really scared that something would happen to their parent, sibling, or family members if they didn't change their eating habits.

Mr. Oliver went to the schools to teach the people who prepare lunches how simple it is to prepare healthy meals. There was much work to be done. For example, he found that the school district considered French fries to be a vegetable on many, if not most, of the days. And the rest of the meal was made up of fried and processed foods, too.

He took the time to show the children how to prepare simple healthy meals and helped them grow a vegetable garden at the school. At one of the schools, he had the children prepare healthy meals for the families so they could taste the new meals the kids had prepared. It was a great success, and everyone, especially the children, enjoyed the healthy meals they had learned to make. Everyone was excited about the changes Mr. Oliver made to the school lunches.

A few months later, he returned to the school to see if they were still serving the healthy meals he had taught them to make.

To his surprise, they were serving the same unhealthy lunches they had been preparing in the past. He was told that the school district said they had to use the ingredients (such as processed foods, unhealthy oils, sugary drinks, and flavored milk) that they were given through the system. Jamie even went to the school district to try to convince them to make the healthy changes. To get kids eating healthier, he launched *Jamie's Home Cooking Skills.* (Seehttp://www.jamieshomecookingskills.com/)

## COMMUNITY CENTERS

Check local community centers in your area and see if they have nutrition classes or classes that teach children how to make healthy food choices. I found a class that taught children to make healthy food choices and taught them how to use a sharp knife properly so they did not get cut when they were slicing vegetables. I did this with my son and taught him how to grow a garden and pick the vegetables and prepare them for dinner. I teach my granddaughters how to make healthy food choices and how to cut fruit and make a healthy sandwich.

Learning to enjoy the taste of real foods is a key to a healthy diet. Teaching your kids to love fruit and vegetables when they first start to eat solid food is essential to creating healthy eating habits that will last a lifetime.

I always teach my granddaughters to make healthy food choices. They will always ask me if something is healthy. I give them healthy snacks and let them help me prepare foods and bake my oat bars. When we are out somewhere together, we never go to a fast food restaurant to eat. I am teaching them by example how to make healthy food choices no matter where they are or what other people are doing. They will know what the healthy choices are for them to eat.

It's interesting to note that the girls also love everything that I cook for them. They eat everything I prepare. (Their favorite has always been salmon with broccoli; it's my favorite, too!)

Children go through a process of learning healthy eating habits. When my granddaughters were ages six and two, I came to visit them and they had a little package of orange Tic-Tacs. The older one gave some to her little sister. They crunched them up three or four at a time until they were gone. Then she looked at me and said, "Are these healthy, Meme?"

I said, "No, they're made out of sugar."

She replied so seriously, "But they are orange, so they must be made with oranges."

I went on to explain to her that it was artificial coloring, sugar, and a lot of chemicals that made them that color and shape, and that make them last a long time on the store shelf. (If you left those on the shelf at home, they'd probably outlast her!) They learned that day to read labels.

Commercials and marketing geared towards children is leading them to think sugary products are good for them. Kids are heavily marketed to because they are easy to persuade and they will bug their parents to have anything that they see on television.

As I have said before, but it bears repeating, television is loaded with unhealthy foods and unhealthy messages that make children think they are eating the best foods in the world. But they are, instead, loaded with sugar, high fructose corn syrup, preservatives, artificial colors, artificial flavors, and additives that make them extremely unhealthy, can lead to many health problems, and may cause their hormones to be thrown off balance.

A good way to combat some of this is to limit your child's access to television. Get them involved in reading books, playing outside, and doing other activities besides sitting in front of the television.

Children will make healthy food choices if parents set a good example and make sure their kids are eating healthy at every meal. Pack a healthy lunch for them every day. Don't have them eat the cafeteria lunch, even if they get it free. School districts consider french fries to be a vegetable. Your child deserves better food to eat than french fries and fried chicken nuggets and other cheap, low-quality foods.

## Experiences with My Son

As a parent, I taught my son how to eat healthy foods and kept him away from sugars. He was a very active baby. I had him tested at UCLA and the doctor told me he was gifted, highly intelligent, and needed to be challenged in school so he would not lose interest. I put him in a private school and found that he did great there.

When my son was in middle school he started having problems sitting still in class. I found out that he was stopping by the store with friends that were buying doughnuts before school. I explained to him that this was not a good choice for him to make. I had to go sit with him in class for the entire day to observe his behavior. That was embarrassing to him and I missed an entire day's work, but that was the teacher's rule with a disruptive student in class. Once we discovered the doughnut problem, my son stopped eating them, and his behavior problems went away.

I heard about a study that was done at one of the schools with students that were always causing problems–getting into fights, skipping classes, and not doing their school work. They were sent to a separate school for problem kids. At this school, they fed the students healthy food for lunch. They did not serve sodas, chocolate milk, cookies, or candy. The lunch was high-quality protein with whole grain bread, plain milk, water, and steamed vegetables, with fruit and yogurt for dessert.

A change was noticed in the behavior of the students immediately. They were not aggressive. They could concentrate in the classroom. And they were happy. When they were interviewed, they said they loved the new meals and didn't feel tired after lunch like they did after lunch at the regular school. They were able to focus on learning instead of getting into trouble. This was a great example of a healthy diet and how all schools should adopt this way of eating.

Children watch what their parents do and what they eat for meals and snacks. It is very important to teach your children to eat healthy and show them that you eat healthy, too. My son and I always ate nutritious foods. Even though I owned my own business and was very busy with work, I always made meals for him instead of buying fast food. I gave him milk to drink instead of juice. We always drank a lot of water. We both still do today!

Learning healthy eating habits at a young age will instill healthy eating habits for life. Children need to drink milk and water, not juice and soda. Teach your children to eat fruit instead of drinking juice. Fruit is loaded with vitamins, fiber, and nutrients their bodies need.

My son always drank milk, not juice, with his meals. We always drank water, and when bottled water came around, it made it easy to carry it around. Refillable bottles are available for your water. We always have a bottle of water with us everywhere we go. My son never saw me without water at hand.

This is an important habit to teach your children. Show them the importance and value of staying hydrated. They need to drink water and milk. They don't need sugary juice or sodas. If they want juice, teach them to eat a juicy orange or any whole fruit. It is loaded with vitamins, fiber, and nutrients that cannot be duplicated; they are only found in nature.

As a parent, you have many responsibilities and teaching your children to eat healthy is one of the most important things you can do. This will set them up for a long and healthy life. One thing you can do to keep your children healthy and avoid obesity, type 2 diabetes and other diseases is to feed your kids healthy meals and teach them to make healthy choices even when you are not around. Temptation is everywhere and just like teaching them to keep away from dangerous situations, it is also important to teach them to stay away from unhealthy foods.

One good habit is to never use food as a reward. When you use food as a reward it gets locked into the brain that good deeds or good behavior will be rewarded with a sugary treat. This sets kids and adults, up for an unhealthy relationship with food. When you give a reward of a book or a game or more time outside being active the right message gets locked into the brain. It is also a great habit to make exercise of any kind a reward. Many people look at exercise as a chore or a punishment. Those are usually the people who end up with problems at a young age or later in life. Activity should always be a treat.

## DESSERTS

Desserts should always be something healthy like fruit, a smoothie made with fruit, air popped popcorn or Skinny Pop or other low-fat no-butter popcorn. For a special treat make some frozen yogurt with fresh berries and plain yogurt with stevia and a banana. This is a treat that is full of nutrients and fiber. Giving your kids cake, candy, chips, dessert, or treats will not give their bodies what they need to grow strong and sugar rots the teeth. If your children learn how to eat healthy meals and snacks, they won't crave sugar if you don't give them sugar. When you serve a nutrient dense meal, the body is full and does not need any more food.

Many times, kids will skimp on eating if they know that a sugary dessert is coming after the meal. By serving healthy meals everyone will feel full and not even think about dessert. If they do feel hungry later, give them some fruit and yogurt or cottage cheese. Milk and turkey have tryptophan that will help them sleep.

It is common knowledge that a doughnut or potato chips is not good for you, and that french fries are full of saturated fats, salt, and calories. Making a healthy version of things the family likes to eat will improve everyone's health. A potato can be microwaved or steamed and cut into the shape of French fries or home fries. Spray a cookie sheet with olive oil or canola cooking spray or wipe the sheet with a paper towel with oil on it and put the potatoes on the cookie sheet. Bake in the oven on broil until they are crispy. I call these my "unfries". They taste like fries without all the fat, and are a perfect alternative to greasy fries or potato chips. Sweet potatoes can be made into "unfries" also which gives another very healthy option. Yams have vitamins and are great to eat with meals and for snacks.

Fast food contains artificial ingredients and sugar along with excess sodium and high fructose corn syrup, MSG, and more preservatives to keep them from going bad. There are so many unhealthy ingredients in fast food that make it an unhealthy option to eat. High Fructose Corn Syrup affects the hormone called ghrelin which tells your brain that you are hungry. When you are full, another hormone called leptin signals your brain to stop eating. (Dr. Oz explains this and more in his book, *The Owner's Manual.*) When you eat HFCS your ghrelin does not shut off and you continue eating even when you are full. This results in eating more food than your body needs, and that causes you to gain weight.

## Baby Foods

The fast food convenience has reached the market for infant foods. There are all types of little snacks that look like freeze-dried foods the astronauts used to eat. There are also little pouches of food instead of food in a jar like I used when my son was a baby. The choices were to make your own baby food by cooking squash and sweet potatoes and mashing them up, which I did all the time. It was cheaper and healthy for my son to eat when he transitioned to baby food. Many parents would us a food processor to make the food smooth and easy for the baby to eat. The other option was to buy the food in the jar.

Today there are so many puffed treats that look like sweetened cereal and do not contain healthy ingredients. Read the labels before buying any baby snacks. The other product that is very popular is the pouch of food. This was meant to be convenient for babies to eat because it could be put on a spoon. It is the consistency of toothpaste. When I read the ingredients it had so many different types of grains, vegetables, milk solids, and yogurt, along with the thickeners that give them a thick consistency. That made me wonder why they are being marketed for babies who are not old enough to drink milk.

I noticed babies being fussy and gassy and also not having normal bowel movements. The babies poop looked like little rocks. Obviously this was not a good food source for a baby that young. Then I noticed people giving the baby the pouch to drink from like a bottle. This is really bad because they are getting too much food at one time. They think it is milk and should be drunk as fast as a bottle. This gives the baby too much food at one time, leading to overweight babies. The baby does not know when to stop eating when they consume food that fast.

I would stick with making your own baby food or using single vegetables and then fruit when you start the baby on solid foods. This gives their tummies time to adjust to eating solid foods and you can also figure out if any of the foods don't agree with the baby. Start with the vegetables that are not sweet to get them used to eating them first. This may be a little less convenient than using a pouch of mixed fruits, vegetables, grains, yogurt, and dairy products, but it is easier for the baby to digest. Your baby will have an easier time getting used to single vegetables at a time than a whole mixture of foods in a pouch. Avoid anything that has preservatives and artificial ingredients in them.

When you spoon feed the baby, it is not only teaching them to eat off a spoon, but it also gives time for the brain to register when the stomach is full. This will slow down the eating and keep the baby from overeating. Good eating habits are also learned in infancy. Take the time to be with your baby and feed them breast milk as long as you can because that is the perfect food for infants.

When it is time to add solid foods, do it gradually and keep track of their bowel movements and fussiness. If they have very hard stool and are fussy they may be getting something that is hard for them to digest. Many of the body's fat cells develop during the first few years of life. Eating the right foods and the right amount is very important for their health.

## THE IMPORTANCE OF EXERCISE

Exercise is so important to everyone and is something that can be done as a family. Take your kids on a walk, a hike, a bike ride, or roller skating. Sitting in the house and playing games on their phones, tablets or computers is keeping kids from getting the exercise they need on a daily basis. Games are addictive and many kids are snacking on junk foods while they play games because they don't want to take time away from the game to eat a healthy meal or any real food. It is easier to play the game and snack on chips. Don't wait until they are overweight or have a health problem. Help your kids understand the importance of eating healthy foods and getting daily exercise. A great way for them to look at what they are eating is to show them the difference between the calories in a slice of pizza and a tuna sandwich or whatever they like to eat. Then teach them how much exercise it takes to burn off those calories extra calories. Show them how to make healthy food choices. That way, when you're not around, they will still know how to eat well.

## MAKE A DIFFERENCE

Make healthy eating and exercise a priority. Plant a garden with your children and let them be involved in growing and picking fresh fruit and vegetables. It is such a great way to get your children interested, active, and making healthy food choices.

If your school does not have a garden, suggest that they start growing one. Suggest the schools start teaching nutrition classes to children. Advocate for healthy meals to be served in the school cafeteria. If this is not possible, make sure you provide your children with a healthy breakfast and a good lunch to take with them.

Lunchables are processed so much so that even the cheese is not real cheese. It is processed cheese. Lunchables contain bologna, mechanically separated chicken, water, pork, corn syrup, modified food starch, contains less than 2% of salt potassium lactate, sodium phosphates, sodiumdiacetate. Sodium ascorbate, flavoring, sodium nitrite, extractives of paprika, potassium phosphate, sugar and potassium chloride. They are convenient, but not a good choice for lunch...for anyone.

You are better off to send hard-boiled eggs and low-fat string cheese, fruit, and plain Greek yogurt. Try a sandwich made with tuna packed in water with relish or Dijon mustard or olive oil mayonnaise or light mayonnaise; nitrate- and hormone-free oven-roasted chicken or turkey or baked tofu. Anything is better than sending processed packaged stuff. Feed your kids real food. You will notice their behavior is better, their skin looks better, and they have more energy. Use healthy bread like Alvarado Street or Ezekiel bread. Even if you use another type of bread that is 100% whole grain and make any type of sandwich it will be better than any prepackaged processed food.

You owe it to your children to eat healthy and exercise daily so you will be around to see them grow up. And you owe it to them to teach them how to eat healthy and exercise daily. No matter what, you are responsible for your children one hundred percent of the time. Planning to feed them healthy meals, wherever they are, is your responsibility, not the school or anyone else. By focusing on healthy eating and daily exercise you can prevent many of the diseases that are being seen in children and keep your kids from becoming obese. Setting a good example is very important and will keep you healthy as well. Kids have enough to worry about without worrying something is going to happen to their parents.

# CHAPTER 10: PUBERTY STARTING VERY EARLY & WAYS TO DELAY ITS START

Teaching your children to eat a healthy diet and to exercise daily is the most important gift you can give to them. Children are exposed to so much sugar, junk food, fast foods, artificial sweeteners and preservatives, along with excess hormones in our food supply that some of them are going into *precocious puberty*. That means they go into puberty before they are ready or should be going into puberty. Some girls as young as seven years old are developing breast buds, one of the signs of early puberty.

This is something that has greatly increased over the past ten years. As I said earlier, one in three kids is obese and children are developing diseases that used to be only encountered by adults. Where are the culprits for this? They are in our food supply and in our homes.

The fast food industry uses a variety of preservatives and flavor enhancers to make food taste better, last longer, and be more appealing to the point of being addictive. The FDA allows hormones (such as estradiol, estriol, testosterone, growth hormone, and progesterone) to be used in our food supply. These hormones can wreak havoc on your bodies and cause children to go into precocious puberty.

Fast foods and junk foods are causing our children to become obese, which leads to increased levels of estrogen in the fat. Children are developing high blood pressure, high cholesterol, type-2 diabetes, and even cancer. The rate of breast cancer can increase with the onset of early puberty. It can also cause the bones to not develop correctly.

Puberty in the past was not starting until early teens, 13 or 14. In many cases children are starting puberty at a very early age. A child who is seven, eight, nine, or even ten years old is not ready for this to happen to them. It is hard enough to deal with when you are a teenager and understand that your body is going to change along with all the other changes puberty brings.

## CAN YOU PREVENT PRECOCIOUS PUBERTY?

There are many things you can do to help prevent precocious puberty, or an early onset of puberty. Eating a healthy diet filled with fresh organic fruits and vegetables with lean proteins that do not have any hormones added will help a lot. Stay away from preservatives, additives, and chemicals that are in processed and packaged foods. Eat as many foods as you can in their natural state and stay away from fast food and junk foods.

Pesticides mimic hormones and should be avoided in your diet. This is easily done by making organic choices at the market and buying produce from local farmers markets. There are also toxins in our shampoos, soaps, and household cleaning products. Parabens are chemicals that are known to create xenoestrogens and can mimic estrogen, contributing to early puberty. Buy organic lotions and shampoo, or at least make sure your products do not contain parabens.

Dr. Jennifer Landa (drjenniferlanda.com [/C:\Users\tracy\AppData\Local\Microsoft\Windows\INetCache\Content.Outlook\M3THZYJ7\drjenniferlanda.com]) recommends preventing precocious puberty by doing the following:

1. Go green—use all organic produce, shop at farmers' markets, and use natural cleaners like baking soda, lemon juice, and vinegar.
2. Become a label reader and avoid products with long words ending in –eth. Avoid products that have parabens, sodium lauryl or lauretha sulfite, triclosan, and triethanolomine or TEA
3. Exercise daily by walking with your family, playing sports, jump rope. Encourage playing sports and go to the park to play tag. Encouraging physical exercise helps a child's

weight management and will further reduce their exposure to hormones.

Eating healthy is the most important thing you can do for yourself and for your children. Make sure that you are doing all that you can to stay healthy so you can be around to take care of your children, making sure they stay healthy and maintain a healthy weight. Work closely with your doctor if your child is experiencing puberty at a very young age. Many doctors are happy to talk to your children about puberty and what to expect. Some parents may have a hard time talking to their children, especially if they are going through puberty at a young age. Knowledge is power and the more you know the better off you and your family will be.

## ENVIRONMENTAL CAUSES

Many chemicals have been banned by the FDA because there is evidence that they disrupt hormone cycles and cause muscle weakness. Triclosan, triclocarbon, and 18 other chemicals found in bath soaps and body washes being marketed, were banned by the FDA. According to npr.org/sections/health [/C:\Users\tracy\AppData\Local\Microsoft\Windows\INetCache\Content.Outlook\M3THZYJ7\npr.org\sections\health] (September 2, 2016), these are used topically, but they are absorbed through the skin. Per the FDA, these products have been banned from use as of September 2, 2016. This was issued by the FDA at the time for immediate release (https://www.fda.gov/newsevents/newsroom/pressannouncements/ucm517478.htm) .

Some research showed that antibacterial washes containing these ingredients are not as effective as plain soap and water and not safe to use long term. These ingredients were banned from being used at this time. Janet Woodcock, M.D., director of the FDA's Center for Drug Evaluation and Research (CDER), said, "In fact, some data suggests that antibacterial ingredients may do more harm than good over the long term." (https://www.usnews.com/news/articles/2016-09-02/fda-says-antibacterial-ingredients-could-do-more-harm-than-good)

Antibacterial active ingredients including triclosan and triclocarban can no longer be added or marketed to consumers. These products include liquid soaps, liquid and foam and gel hand soap, bar soap, and body washes. Triclosan is also added to certain clothing, cookware, furniture, and toys to reduce and prevent bacterial contamination, but these are not regulated by the FDA. The study has raised questions about whether triclosan is hazardous to human health. Researchers found triclosan alters hormone regulators in animals and contributes to development of antibiotic-resistant germs and might be harmful to the immune system.

A study designed to test the amount of triclosan exposure took urine samples from adults and children in 2008 and found 75% contained triclosan (https://www.ncbi.nlm.nih.gov/pmc/ articles/PMC2265044/ ). Triclosan is not an essential ingredient. It may help prevent gingivitis when added to toothpaste, but there is no evidence that antibacterial soaps and body wash are more effective than regular soap in preventing illness or the spread of certain diseases, according to the FDA.

Make sure your children are using natural products and avoid BPA plastics. Never reheat food in a plastic container or put hot food into a plastic container or bag. Clean your home with natural products such as vinegar, lemon juice, and baking soda. These are much cheaper and much safer for your family. Avoid products that are scented. Taking care to do these things will help keep your family from being exposed to dangerous chemicals that can cause illness and hormone problems.

The bottom line is that we as parents and grandparents owe it to our children to educate them in the importance of eating a healthy diet. It makes sense to avoid all chemicals, preservatives, artificial colors and flavorings, and the hormones in meats and other products. This is a lot of information for an overall view of some of the problems with foods and products used daily. Do the best you can to protect your family from chemicals and always eat a healthy diet.

# CHAPTER 11: IMPORTANCE OF DRINKING WATER & AVOIDING SUGARY DRINKS

## HOW I STAY HYDRATED

Every morning when I wake up, I drink a full glass of room-temperature water with the juice from half of a lemon. I go to the gym with a large bottle of water that I drink throughout my workout. I do cardiovascular exercise and lift weights.

If I stay home to exercise I drink a full bottle of water during my workout. I have a water bag that I wear when I ride my bike outside. The water bag makes it easy to drink while I am riding. I have another water bag that I can wear if I am walking or hiking. I never drink sodas or sports drinks, and I avoid alcohol. When I get home, I drink more water and continue drinking water all day long.

In Japan, it is customary to drink two or three glasses of water first thing in the morning to start the day. The liver is very active at night and the body is working very hard to repair itself. This is part of why that first glass of water is so important in the morning.

Besides adding a nice flavor to the water, lemon also helps to stimulate stomach digestion and bile production. It contains vitamin C and potassium. A German study found that drinking water, especially lemon water, helps increase metabolism and aids in maintaining a healthy weight.

Drink water frequently throughout the day. Drinking a glass of water before a meal will help reduce the amount of food you eat. Dehydration can be mistaken for hunger. Staying well hydrated helps hold hunger at bay. Don't wait until you feel thirsty to drink water because that means you are already dehydrated.

Thirst is a sign of dehydration. If you wait until you feel thirsty to drink water you have already waited too long. Drinking water before you feel thirsty will keep you hydrated and keep you from feeling hungry when you are thirsty.

## ARTIFICIAL SWEETENERS

Most doctors will tell you that sodas are not good for adults or children. Soda is not good for your teeth, and whether sweetened with sugar or artificially sweetened, they are not a healthy beverage choice. There is nothing nutritionally available for your body in soda. When the body is given artificial ingredients, it does not recognize them and cannot use them.

Artificial sweetener has been shown to increase cravings for sugar because it is sweeter than sugar. Reports on artificial sweetener have shown that people who drink diet sodas end up gaining more weight. Because it is sweeter than sugar, this causes the body to not properly recognize sweetness.

According to Harvard's T.H. Chan School of Public Health, a 2013 study showed that drinking soda sweetened with sugar and soda with artificial sweetener are both linked to a risk of developing type-2 diabetes. (https://www.hsph.harvard.edu/nutritionsource/healthy-drinks/artificial-sweeteners/) Another study of 3,682 people found a relationship between using drinks with artificial sweeteners and weight gain. Participants in this study were followed for seven or eight years, and their weight was monitored, taking into consideration their diet, exercise changes, and diabetes status. They found that those using artificial sweetener had an increase of 47% in their BMI (body mass index), more than those who did not drink artificial sweeteners.

## WHAT ABOUT COFFEE AND TEA?

Coffee is a popular beverage that gets a lot of attention because so many people drink it. Coffee has caffeine and is addicting. People who use coffee every day may experience headaches or feel tired if they don't have their coffee.

Coffee in high doses can raise your levels of epinephrine, known as adrenaline. This can increase blood pressure. There are claims that a cup of coffee each day is good for the heart, but you will need to make that decision on your own. If you have any heart problems, consult your doctor before using any type of caffeine or another stimulant.

Some claims have been made that organic coffee is better for you to drink. I like to recommend going all organic, but if you don't drink much coffee and are following my healthy eating plan, the choice is up to you. If caffeine makes you jittery, I say it is probably best to stay away from coffee or caffeine or at least limit the amount you consume.

Coffee speeds up the heart rate, but regular coffee drinkers build up a tolerance for it. I have been told by nurses who work in post-operation facilities that the heart can have an irregular beat for a few minutes if you are a regular coffee drinker. They also notice their coffee drinking patients tend to have headaches when they don't get their caffeine.

Specialty coffee drinks can have a lot of calories, especially when they contain chocolate, whipped cream, caramel, or any other flavorings. Those extra calories add up fast! A coffee drink can be between 300 – 500 calories. That's enough calories for an entire meal.

While fancy coffee drinks are often loaded up with sugars and fats, even using cream and sugar in your regular coffee increases the number of calories and fat. By comparison, a cup of black coffee has only a few calories. Using a little non-fat milk to lighten it up and adding a little bit of stevia instead of sugar and cream will keep you calories from a cup of coffee very low.

This is a good place to add this note about stevia and sweeteners. I carry packets of stevia in my purse so I always have a healthy substitute for sugar handy. And having it on hand keeps the artificial sweeteners away, too.

Some health food stores have packets at their coffee counters. Some places like Starbucks have their first stevia-based sweetener which has stevia and monk fruit, a sweetener derived from dried fruit. They claim it is a zero-calorie product and safe for pregnant women and for children as well as diabetics and those wishing to reduce their calorie intake.

I recommend that you read the packaging. I prefer to use packets that contain only pure stevia leaf, but you will find some that are partly sugar or partly artificial sweetener, too. Some other names for sugar are sucrose, dextrose, fructose, and high fructose corn syrup (the worst one that you should always avoid).

Tea comes in many different varieties, and some even help you relax. Chamomile tea is good to drink when you want to unwind at the end of the day. It has a very mild taste and does not have any caffeine. Green tea is another good option that comes with benefits. On webmd.com, it says that green tea, in the brain, blocks the formation of plaques linked to Alzheimer's (https://www.webmd.com/alzheimers/news/20050920/antioxidant-in-green-tea-may-fight-alzheimers).

Tea can be served hot or cold. It makes a great option for people who choose not to drink coffee. Green tea does have some caffeine, but not as much as coffee or black tea. Stevia is a great sweetener for tea as well.

Green tea has been shown to have beneficial properties and can be found in tea bags so you can steep it yourself at home and make either hot or iced tea. Tea has only two calories if you don't add any milk or sugar. Black tea has more caffeine than green tea and both are great to drink instead of coffee. There are also many herbal teas that taste great and do not have any caffeine.

## WHAT DOES TRACY DO?

When I was younger, I hated the smell of coffee and had no desire to drink or even taste it. My parents drank coffee, but I never wanted to even try it. As an adult, I used to drink iced tea and sometimes hot tea, but not on a consistent basis. Water has always been my favorite drink.

As a kid the only time we drank sodas was when we went camping in Yosemite National Park for two weeks every summer. It is a beautiful place. I loved being there and swimming in the river. Back then you could drink the water right out of the river. I loved the taste of fresh spring water. I still drink natural alkaline spring water or filtered water.

My husband, as with most people in the Army, learned to drink black coffee made in a big container large enough for all the troops. For our anniversary, I bought him a Nespresso Coffeemaker. Sometimes I drink a little decaffeinated coffee. When we are traveling I sometimes share a non-fat latte with my husband. But on a daily basis, the only thing I need to drink is water.

## ALCOHOL

Alcoholic beverages contain a lot of calories that add to your daily calorie count if you choose to drink alcohol. Alcohol also slows down your metabolism which means you do not burn as many calories as you would if you were not drinking alcohol. According to the American Cancer Society, "Drinking more than a glass a day of alcohol contributes to the risk of breast cancer in both men and women, and it also impairs your judgment." It is very hard to make good decisions if you are drinking alcohol.

The number of calories in an alcoholic beverage varies depending on the type of drink. One margarita can have 500 calories per glass. Mixes for alcohol drinks have a lot of sugar, artificial flavors, and even artificial colors.

Many drinks have sugar or salt on the rim of the glass they are served in. Maraschino cherries in drinks are loaded with sugar and artificial ingredients. Fresh cherries are great to eat, but avoid the maraschino cherries.

Beer has about 154 calories per glass and a pint of Guinness beer has 170 calories. A glass of wine has 124 calories in a five-ounce serving. One bottle of wine has about 644 calories. Dry white wine has about 85 calories in a 125-ml glass. No matter what type of alcohol you drink, the amount of calories will add up fast and lead to weight gain.

Alcohol will cause weight gain in your abdomen, and for women, it will also increase your bottom size. The bottom line is, drinking alcohol will add extra calories and cause weight gain. If you get into a daily habit of drinking, it can cause problems and illnesses as well as contribute to obesity and increase your risk for cancer. Even a few drinks a week has been linked to an increase of breast cancer in women.

The American Cancer Society also says that risks of cancer of the throat, esophagus, mouth, liver, colon, rectum, and breast have been linked to alcohol use. Drinking and smoking together clearly raises the risk of cancers more than either drinking or smoking alone. (https://www.cancer.org/cancer/cancer-causes/diet-physical-activity-alcohol-use-and-cancer.html)

Many accidents and deaths have been caused by people who drive under the influence of alcohol. A comedian once said that a vehicle is basically a weapon that you drive. People who drink and drive run the risk of hurting themselves or other people. Many fights occur because people are drinking, and some of them result in serious injuries. Many deaths are linked to drinking and driving. If you drink, don't drive.

At social occasions drink sparkling water and a splash of juice with a twist of lemon or lime. It looks like you are drinking; no one needs to know it is water. When reducing the amount of alcohol, switch to half wine or champagne with half juice or sparkling water. This literally can cut the number of calorie of your drink in half. It also cuts the amount of alcohol you are consuming. By putting less alcohol and more sparkling water in your glass, you can stop drinking alcohol. Having an occasional glass of wine will be a better option than a nightly habit.

When making a choice about drinking alcohol, consider the fact that a glass of alcohol can have as many calories as a chicken breast, steamed broccoli, and brown rice. Would you rather have a healthy meal and feel good all night and the next day or drink alcohol? The choice will be easier when you look at it this way.

If you are having trouble losing weight or are continuing to gain weight, look at the additional calories you may be drinking. Remember that alcohol not only has a lot of calories, but it also slows down your metabolism which causes you to burn fewer calories.

Drinking alcohol also lowers inhibitions, which makes you feel braver and more relaxed. In this condition, making healthy food choices becomes more difficult. So, if you must drink alcohol, limit yourself to one day a week or one drink. If you get into a daily habit of drinking, it can cause problems and illnesses as well as contribute to obesity and increase your risk for cancer.

## YOU DECIDE...

When deciding what beverages to drink, make water your first choice. Every function in your body requires water. Giving your body enough water to function well will help you feel great. And there are no calories or artificial ingredients in it!

Some flavored waters do have artificial sweeteners and other ingredients. Check the labels of any drinks that are not clear or that have flavors added. I recommend that you avoid everything with added sugar, artificial ingredients, and preservatives. There are some bottled waters that have natural flavors. These are fine to drink as long as they don't have sugar added. I enjoy drinking Pellegrino or Perrier sparkling water when I go out for dinner. Sparkling water is a great choice.

# CHAPTER 12: How to Eat When You Travel

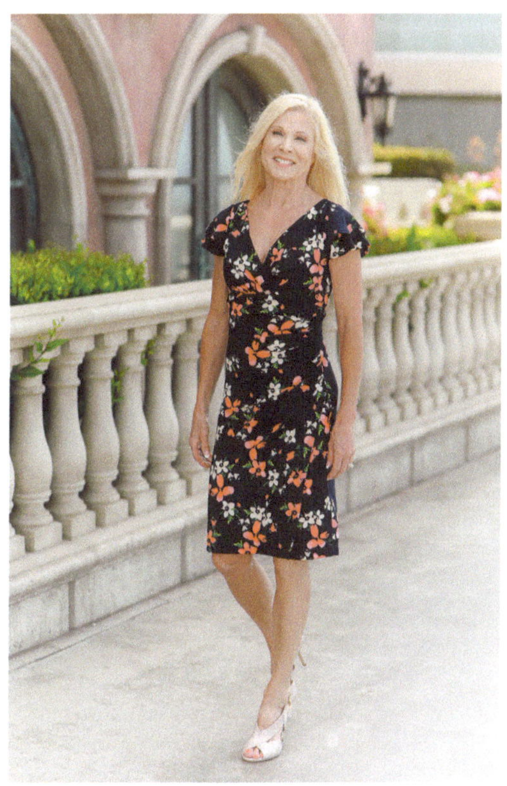

There is never a time when you cannot eat healthy, regardless of where you are. Even when you travel, you can still find a way to eat healthy. It just takes planning and keeping your healthy focus.

When you travel, you adjust what you bring to eat depending on the mode of travel.

### WHAT TO BRING ON THE AIRPLANE

There are very strict rules about what you can bring on an airliner. The Transportation Security Administration (TSA) will not let you bring liquids, water, or yogurt. Sandwiches are usually no problem to bring on a plane. I make tofu or chicken sandwiches and some steamed Japanese yams. I usually make date-nut bread if we are traveling across the country which is convenient when delayed on a plane. I used to bring squash and cauliflower dishes on the plane, but with the new rules on what you can take on with you, it is easier to bring something that is readily identifiable to the TSA. When you bring your own food, it makes traveling by plane less stressful, especially if you get delayed or your flight is canceled.

Once you arrive at your location it is easy to find good food to eat especially if you are going to some place like Los Angeles where there are many healthy options. Many restaurants have gluten free meals which usually don't have any sauces on them. Ordering your food plain without any butter, oil, or seasoning is the best way to insure it is all healthy with no fatty sauces, oils, or flavor enhancers like Monosodium Glutamate (MSG).

When you order your food, always ask them to prepare your food without any butter, oil, or seasoning. Get vinegar for your salad instead of fatty salad dressing and skip the bread and butter. If you are hungry when you arrive ask for a salad. Most appetizers are fried or not very healthy, but you can always get a salad or shrimp cocktail. Either one is healthier than eating the bread and butter or the usual appetizer (unless they specialize in healthy appetizers, of course).

I went to a restaurant for a work-related dinner with Jerry and some people we had never met before. I was starving and wanted to order food, but everyone else ordered appetizers. I ordered a salad for my appetizer. As it turned out, one of the appetizers was a tower of shrimp and lobster. Since it was steamed and not prepared with butter, I could eat that, too. By the time my dinner came, I was already full, so I ended up bringing it back to the hotel and sharing it with Jerry the next day for lunch.

Which brings me to another travel tip: always get a hotel room with a refrigerator. Make sure the temperature is set so your food will stay cold but does not freeze. If you can get a room with a refrigerator, stovetop, and microwave, you can make an endless number of meals in your room. This saves a lot of money by not eating at a restaurant for all your meals.

Tuna comes in convenient pouches that are great to take when you are on the go or when you have a flight to catch. If I am just going to work or have an appointment, I put my tuna in Tupperware and put it in my lunch with a cold pack. Then I can sit in the car and eat or find a store that has tables outside or inside when it's cold.

Some stores make brown rice sushi with ahi tuna and avocado or a vegetable roll with tuna. Brown rice is more nutritious and it tastes great. They also have rice paper vegetable rolls with shrimp or tofu. Some have vegetarian rolls. Organic food stores are great places to find a quick healthy lunch or take-home for dinner. I love being in southern California because you can be outside all year long. Who needs seasons when you have great weather all year? Yes, I am a California girl through and through.

## CONVENTIONS

Traveling for work often means going to a convention where there is a set menu or two choices of entrée. Any convention or banquet has a menu that you can special order in advance and sometimes even the night of the event. Many people eat gluten-free or vegetarian meals which are usually available, but try to order plain chicken or fish in advance. Usually you can request no butter, oil, or seasoning, and you will get a great healthy meal. Another option is to order a plain salad and bring a chicken breast or tofu with you to put on top. I used to do this before I figured out I could call and speak with the food service manager and make a special request for a meal prepared the way I want it. With a healthy meal to eat it takes the stress out of picking through whatever mystery meat is on your plate and worrying about what you are eating. Many people have special diets these days, so it is not uncommon for people to call ahead and order gluten-free, vegetarian meals, or even order fish or chicken instead of beef.

My homemade oat bars are always with me when I go places. If a meeting runs long or I am at a doctor's appointment I can eat a few oat squares to hold me over until lunch. They are great meal replacement bars. I created this recipe when my first granddaughter was born. We make them together and now her sisters eat them too. These oat squares have saved my husband during a long meeting and me when I am stuck in traffic. If I am at a buffet and they forget my meal, I go to the buffet and fill my plate with fruit, vegetables and salad with no dressing. I can put some oat bars that are cut into squares on my plate along with some tofu. This way I always have a plate with food on it so no one asks why I am not eating. In the past, I would put my food on my plate and swap plates with my husband when he finished eating.

Speaking with managers and staff about healthy options for meals is a good way to bring about changes in what foods are served at banquets. Healthy meals should always be an option and I hope they become the standard. When you preorder a healthy meal make sure to let people know that healthy meals are greatly appreciated. Make the managers and the staff feel good about serving healthy foods.

When ordering your food at a restaurant, asking for it with no butter, oil, or seasoning also insures that your meal has no high fructose corn syrup, sugar, or MSG. It is very important to tell your server to make sure your food is prepared the way you ordered it. There are not too many places where you cannot get your food cooked to order unless they are a premade meal in which case you special order your food in advance.

## STAYING AT A HOTEL

Staying at a hotel can be very expensive and stressful unless you plan ahead. Choose a hotel chain and stay in the same hotel or one of their partner hotels when you travel so you can earn points towards a free nights or free breakfast.

If you are in a hotel with a microwave, refrigerator, and some kind of stovetop, it is very easy to save hundreds of dollars that you would spend eating every meal in restaurants. In order to do this, find a healthy store like Whole Foods, or any other store that carries organic produce and Ezekiel bread. Buy some fresh organic vegetables, raw carrots, canned or packaged tuna or chicken breast along with fresh fish. Lettuce is always great to use as a top for open-faced sandwiches. You will have enough food for lunch and dinner.

Some hotels have a full restaurant that serves breakfast, lunch, and dinner and others just serve breakfast. Many hotels have a buffet with a lot of pastries and bagels which you should avoid. If the hotel has free breakfasts, choose wisely and get oatmeal, hard-boiled eggs, or scrambled egg whites with one yolk (no butter, oil, or seasonings). Don't get an omelet unless they can make it without oil. They usually put one or two scoopers of oil in the pan before they cook the omelet so it won't stick. Ask for the eggs to be made in a pan with just a little cooking spray. Add any vegetables they have. Having crispy vegetables in your scrambled eggs gives you some added flavor and crunch. Look for eggs, egg whites, oatmeal and fresh fruit. This will be a nutritious breakfast, and it will save you money. I order egg whites prepared this way or get hard boiled eggs. I bring a yam or a slice of my Ezekiel bread to eat with my eggs.

Another good thing to do is find a store and buy Ezekiel Bread, rice cheese, seasoned tofu or tuna so you can make some sandwiches for lunch. When we are at a convention where there is not going to be a store close by, I grill chicken breasts to bring with me. It saves a lot of money when you can prepare some of your meals and get free breakfast.

I use the chicken breasts and tofu to make sandwiches for lunch so we can take them with us, no matter where we go. Many times, we are in a meeting or on someone else's schedule and I get hungry. I always have food with me so my blood sugar does not get too low and my oat bars have saved me every time.

## Be Prepared

When we travel across the country, it is always an adventure. I plan our food on the day before we are scheduled to leave, making either sandwiches with tofu, mustard, and lettuce or a grilled chicken breast with mustard and lettuce on Ezekiel Sesame bread. I make my husband a whole sandwich and an open-faced sandwich for myself. I always make a few extra sandwiches so that if we get delayed or our flight gets canceled, we don't have to search for food or eat fast food at the airport. I bring my famous oat bars and my famous date or banana bread along with a Japanese yam. If we have apples or grapes at home, I bring some fruit, too.

I am always prepared with a quick easy meal. If the day runs long, the extra sandwiches can be our dinner. If we don't eat the sandwiches that day, we eat them for lunch the next day.

## TRAVELLING WITH CHILDREN

Help your children choose healthy foods when traveling like oatmeal, wheat toast, eggs, and milk instead of juice. If you let them load up on sugar at breakfast they will be climbing the walls in the hotel. Then the sugar crash comes and they are tired and grouchy. By teaching your kids to eat healthy no matter where they are they will learn to eat healthy when you're not around. This is a learning process for kids and is very important for them to know. If you teach your children at a young age to choose whole foods, whole grains, and fruits and vegetables instead of sugary cereal and junk foods, it will make their lives and yours much easier.

If you are making a change in your family because you have been eating junk and fast foods, be sure to explain to your family why you are making this change. Let your children know that you want them to grow up healthy and strong, eating a healthy diet and exercising to achieve optimum health. Many children will join the team and your whole family will benefit.

Whether you are traveling with your family or going on a work trip, the plan is still the same. Bring food with you and suggest that co-workers do the same. If you have food and your co-worker or travel companion does not, you will still waste time looking for food when you arrive. Help your friends and family by suggesting they bring food with them, and give them simple guidelines for what to bring–or just tell them to buy my book.

When my granddaughters travel with me, I bring food and water for them. I make sure not to give them any sugar. We make my oat bars along with sandwiches and pack fruit for the trip. When we are going to take a flight, we prepare our food the day before. We buy water at the airport before boarding our flight. Buying water before boarding is important because I have been on flights that have run out of drinking water. If the flight is delayed from taking off and we are stuck on the plane longer than expected, we are prepared.

It does not take more than five minutes to make a sandwich if you have followed my shopping guide and have food on the shelf, in the refrigerator, or in the freezer to use. If you don't want to use any bread, bring along some baked or steamed yams, squash, or baked potato and baked tofu or grilled chicken.

I flew across the country to be with son, his wife, and my granddaughters. We met up, then drove to Monterey where we rented a house on the beach for a few days. We expected to stay at that house and not go anywhere else. I brought chicken breasts and Ezekiel bread with me. I also brought organic egg whites and tomatoes for breakfasts and some Yukon Gold potatoes that could be used for breakfast or dinner. The kids love teriyaki tofu which is great for making sandwiches to bring along.

I made two chicken breast sandwiches for the drive to Monterey which was two hours away from where my son lives. We arrived too early to check into the house immediately. Everyone else was scrambling for fast food except us because we had our chicken breast sandwiches and tofu. I had fruit and tofu for the kids. Simple planning made the trip much easier.

You can throw together a salad or thaw out some lentil soup faster than you can decide what fast food to eat. Convenience is the key to being successful improving your health and losing that extra weight you have been carrying around. Planning ahead is a definite winning key for traveling and eating healthy at the same time.

I have been traveling around the world for decades, and I have never been in a situation where I resorted to fast food because that was all there was to eat. Planning is the key to success. If you plan to succeed, you will. If you fail to plan, you plan to fail. If you think it is hard to eat healthy, you are choosing not to eat healthy. If you follow my easy shopping tips and my healthy meals in minutes, you will be successful at eating healthy, losing weight easily, and greatly improving your health and energy level.

# CHAPTER 13: HOLIDAY HEALTHY MEALS & SURVIVING THE HOLIDAYS

Holidays are always a very challenging time of year because of all the parties and holiday foods. Holidays make it easy to go off your healthy eating plan and just give in to temptation. If you indulge on one day it won't take away all the good you have done by changing to this healthy eating plan. But when you start eating candy at Halloween and continue until Thanksgiving and then through Christmas until the end of the year, you will start off the New Year with extra pounds to lose. The most popular New Year's Resolution is to lose weight. The problem is that most people gain weight over the holidays and never lose it.

My solution is my healthy eating plan. If you follow this plan all year long it won't matter if you overeat on one day. If you are very active you may get away with doing this a few times a year, but if you make it a habit of overeating or eating unhealthy foods the pounds will start adding up, and before you know it, your weight is out of control.

Therefore, make healthy food choices a priority every day of the year. On the holidays follow my easy calorie cutting tips and it won't matter if you eat a little more on one or two days a year. There are many ways to cut calories over the holidays and every calorie counts. With all the high fat foods served at Thanksgiving, Christmas, and New Year's Eve, it is important to start planning early.

## HEALTHY HOLIDAY OPTIONS

Learn how to make healthy low-fat meals and enjoy your holiday feast. The white meat of the turkey is from the breast and that is low in fat–a good lean protein. Get a turkey that is organic or at least make sure it has not been injected with butter and oils. Don't use additional butter or oil on the turkey, and if you stuff the turkey, find a healthy recipe for dressing that isn't loaded with butter and oil. I suggest cooking dressing separately so it does not get the greasy drippings from the turkey making your dressing lower in fat.

Make your yams steamed, not candied with butter and brown sugar. That just adds calories and fat to a delicious low-calorie yam. You can use stevia for baking if you really feel a need to sweeten a "sweet potato."

Yukon Gold potatoes are less starchy and make great mashed potatoes. Fix them without butter or cream. Use a little non- or low-fat milk or even some of the water from the potatoes. You can also bake the potatoes or cook them in the microwave, then mash them. Add a Japanese yam to your potatoes or just use mashed Japanese yams instead of potatoes. They are very buttery and creamy tasting and make a great "mashed potato" that is sweet and creamy.

Add some cauliflower to your potatoes by mashing it in with them. If your family will eat cauliflower and broccoli put them on the side for them to eat. Fill your plate with half vegetables, a quarter for starchy vegetables and a quarter for turkey.

I have a recipe for healthy baked beans (see chapter 18). Beans are full of fiber and are good for you to eat. However, when you add a lot of sugar and molasses, salt and pork they become very high in calories and fat. Modify the recipe to make it low in sugar and use turkey bacon instead of ham or salt pork or make vegetarian beans.

Vegetables can be mixed vegetables, corn, cauliflower, and broccoli. I like to always serve a cruciferous vegetable with my meals because they help fight cancer. Make a beautiful salad full of a variety of vegetables such as spinach, red cabbage, tomatoes, artichoke hearts, kidney and garbanzo beans. Many people go back for seconds or want to eat more. Salad fills you up and it is okay to go back for seconds. Use the flavor of the beans and vegetables instead of fatty salad dressing or use balsamic vinegar.

If you make gravy use only a small amount of drippings from the turkey and use an organic or healthy turkey gravy mix to cut down on the amount of fat you are eating. Use gravy very sparingly. Some people pour gravy over everything which creates a very high-fat and high-calorie meal. Sticking with what I have given you so far keeps your meal very healthy. If you are eating beans, use the juice from the beans as your gravy. Put your beans on top of your potatoes or yams instead of gravy.

## Healthy Holiday Desserts

Dessert can also be made healthy by cutting the calories when you make pumpkin pie. Use low- fat canned milk and make a healthy pie crust out of nuts or whole grain flour, or don't use a crust at all. If you are eating out for a meal, skip the pie or just have a small piece and don't eat the crust. Skip the whipped cream which is full of fat and sugar.

If you are eating healthy all the time, it won't hurt you to eat a piece of pumpkin pie for Thanksgiving. If you eat the filling and not the crust or the whipped cream, it is actually not that bad. The pumpkin is good for you and if you make the pie yourself you can use stevia, xylitol, low-fat canned milk, and spices. The pie will have less fat, fewer calories, and be good for you.

(Crust is usually Crisco, butter, and white flour, which is basically glue.)

Using whole wheat or an oat flour crust along with nuts, applesauce, or another healthy option will give you a better tasting and healthier crust. Many times, I don't even use a pie crust. I make a banana cream pie from vanilla pudding and bananas topped with egg whites and xylitol made into meringue. This is much healthier than a store-bought pie and it tastes great. I can make a crust out of nuts, a little butter, and applesauce.

I have a recipe for a crust made with walnuts and one that is made from oat flour, but to me crust is just extra calories that you don't need. Eat the pie filling and leave the fatty crust behind so it does not end up on your behind.

Surviving the holidays will not be hard if ask yourself if what you are eating is good for you. Is this food nutritious or is it just something you want because it is sweet? If you think you are going to crave something sweet, make a special treat like banana bread using stevia and xylitol instead of sugar and use oat flour instead of white flour. This is a good way to cut calories and make a healthier treat.

You can do this with everything that you make and everything you eat. Cut calories by using stevia and/or xylitol and use egg whites instead of whole eggs or one whole egg and two egg whites. If the recipe calls for nuts, reduce the amount of nuts down from a cup or half cup to a third or even a quarter cup and chop up the nuts so they are distributed throughout the bread or whatever you are planning to bake.

Make a fruit salad or a fruit cup with yogurt and berries and layer it with plain Greek yogurt, berries, nuts, and seeds. This makes a great parfait and is the perfect dessert. There are many great fruits that really keep you from craving sugar, especially if you eat them with plain yogurt.

Persimmons are one of my favorite fruits. They are a winter fruit and are very sweet and delicious. If you have not tried them you should. Look for a farmers market that sells them. They are cheaper than buying them at the store. They can be eaten when they are soft or eaten when they are hard. The ones that are shaped like an acorn need to be either peeled or have the inside fruit scooped out. These are very good if you freeze them and let them thaw out just enough to scoop out the frozen insides. It is like a very sweet sorbet, but tastes better and is full of fiber and vitamins.

Baked goods can be made with fewer calories and less sugar by always choosing the low-fat and low- or no-sugar versions of everything. Sweeten everything with Stevia Leaf, Truvia, or xylitol instead of sugar. I have made so many different types of desserts, even a low-fat no-sugar cheesecake that everyone loved. Pumpkin pie, pecan pie, and banana cream pie can all be made in a low-fat, low-sugar version that saves a lot of calories.

This does not mean that you can eat several pieces or eat the whole thing. Stick to one thin slice and even split it with someone. I cut my cheesecake in little squares and put each piece in a cupcake paper and sent it to work with my husband along with some forks. Everyone has a great treat which I made healthier by substituting ingredients and using low-fat cream cheese and stevia and xylitol.

There are always ways of making any meal and even desserts healthier. The trick with desserts is to limit them to special occasions and make them nutritious. By making fruit and yogurt desserts or homemade pudding that is low in fat and sugar-free you can have your dessert. When making dessert for a special occasion, cut calories by using my suggestions and limit the amount to a very small piece or share it with someone. It's even good to skip the pies, cakes, and cookies altogether. Have fresh berries and Greek yogurt instead. This is always a big hit and when you put it in a parfait the presentation makes it look and taste special. It is the perfect snack or dessert.

Surviving the holidays without feeling deprived is very easy if you plan your meals and stick with the healthy eating plan. Holidays can be both fun and healthy.

# CHAPTER 14: REDUCING STRESS

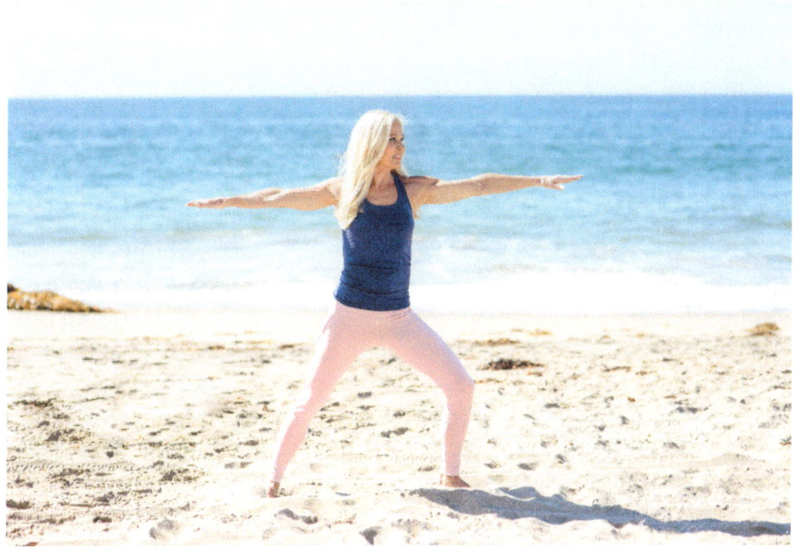

Stress is something that everyone has in their life to varying degrees. People look at stress and deal with it in different ways. If you take two people and put them under the same stress they will react differently.

There are times in our lives when a little voice tells us to do something or lets us know that something is wrong. Listen to that voice and make changes in your life. When you eat a poor diet and don't get any exercise you will feel tired and sluggish. If you are under more stress than your body can handle, things start breaking down. You can become ill from too much stress.

A little stress is good because it can motivate you to work harder or make changes to relieve some of the stress. But when the stress starts causing problems, it is time to look at your life to see how you can change it for the better.

One of the most helpful habits you can learn is to always be aware of your own stress levels. Recognizing this is the first step in getting a handle on it and making changes that will lower the pressure and avoid the stress-related problems.

There are some stressful situations that commonly effect people in the same way. A tax audit is a good example. No one likes to be audited and I think most people will be a little stressed out if they find themselves in that process.

Other stressful situations (such as driving in traffic) affect people differently. One person may turn on an audio book or relaxing music while another will get enraged and start yelling and honking the horn. Someone else may feel stressed, but tries to hold the bad feelings inside. Everyone has their own way of dealing with stress, and it usually depends on what the stress is.

Stress or being nervous can cause one person to jump up and go for a run and then come back to deal with the stressful situation after they feel calm. Stress may be the reason someone starts their own business. But when people deal with stress by doing unhealthy things like overeating or using drugs or alcohol it is time to turn that behavior around. The person who is using food as a way to deal with stress has not figured out other ways of dealing with pressure. There are a number of healthy ways to deal with stress, and it is important to learn some of those ways.

## Symptoms and Effects of Stress

According to the Mayo Clinic, stress symptoms can affect your body, your thoughts and feelings, and your behavior. Being able to recognize common stress symptoms can give you a jump on managing them. Stress left unchecked can contribute to many health problems such as high blood pressure, heart disease, obesity, and diabetes. (April 28, 2016 https://www.mayoclinic.org/healthy-lifestyle/stress-management/in-depth/stress-symptoms/art-20050987).

The Mayo Clinic has Healthy Lifestyle Stress Management information. Stress can affect your health in ways you might not realize. The site says you may think it is an illness which is giving you a headache, frequent insomnia, or decreased productivity at work. But stress can be the culprit. Being able to recognize stress will give you a jump on managing it. (https://www. mayoclinic.org/healthy-lifestyle/stress-management/basics/stress-basics/hlv-20049495)

One thing that stress does is trigger a release of cortisol. Cortisol has a direct impact on the whole hormonal system. I am sure you have heard the commercials about how high cortisol levels lead to belly fat. High levels of cortisol cause many problems with thyroid hormones, blood sugar hormones (insulin), and sex hormones (progesterone, estrogen, and testosterone).

Stress uses up the body's natural hormones and leaves their levels low.

Most women don't have hormone issues while on vacation because they are relaxing on a beach and not stressing. This makes them feel better. Stress causes the body to use up its natural hormones and leaves the body lower of vital hormones. Stress affects your body's ability to create the feel-good hormone, serotonin.

Common effects of stress on your body are

- Headache
- Muscle tension or pain
- Chest pain
- Fatigue
- Changes in sex drive
- Stomach upset
- Sleep problems

Common effects of stress on your moods are:

- Anxiety
- Restlessness
- Lack of motivation or focus
- Feeling overwhelmed
- Irritability or anger
- Sadness or depression

Common effects of stress on your behavior are:

- Overeating or under-eating

- Angry outbursts
- Drug or alcohol abuse
- Tobacco use
- Social withdrawal
- Exercising less often

Taking steps to manage stress can have numerous health benefits. Explore stress management strategies such as

- Regular physical activity
- Relaxation techniques such as deep breathing, meditation, or yoga
- Tai Chi or getting a massage
- Keeping a sense of humor
- Socializing with family and friends
- Setting aside time for hobbies such as reading a book or listening to music

## How I Handle Stress

My husband and I love to do everything together. When you have someone you love to be with it makes life great. He does not let stress get to him and he is always positive and calm. His parents were the same way and it was always great to be around them and to talk to them because they were always happy. My husband is the same way which makes him a pleasure to be around.

I did not grow up with the same type of parents. I had to learn on my own how to deal with stress and how to be a positive person. Being positive is a great way to reduce stress. Just planning the future without any fears and knowing that no matter what, everything is going to work out great will make you feel calm and reduce stress.

One of the things I like to do is write down all the things that give me joy and can change my moods immediately. Exercise is at the top of the list for me. Going to the gym is a great stress reliever. Lifting weights and using the elliptical trainer and other equipment are helpful. Other things I enjoy are writing in a journal or on my computer, reading a book, going for a walk, doing floor exercises and working on my reformer at home, watching a movie with my husband, doing something nice for someone else, baking bread, calling or sending cards to friends, and visiting them.

One of the best ways to feel better fast is to do a random act of kindness. I buy a big package of food and snacks, then drive around looking for people in need and give them a treat. This is something that I never do alone and I make sure I am in a safe area. Sometimes I will just leave something with a note on a bench or somewhere where I have seen homeless or less fortunate people.

Calling my granddaughters on Skype is one of my favorite things to do. It is not as good as seeing them in person, but it gives them a chance to talk to me and see me at the same time. It is magical to be able to see them thousands of miles away on my computer. The little one thinks we are behind her computer screen and will always look behind it, trying to find us there. The middle one loves to tell us what she is doing and make pictures for us. The oldest just got a medal for reading more books than anyone else in school. She loves a challenge and will do everything she can to reach her goal. (This is a characteristic to have and to nurture.) Children are pure joy and they are so easy to entertain. They love to be silly and do funny things. This is a great thing to draw out of yourself—that silly side of you that wants to laugh and have fun. Joy is being fun-loving and curious like a child.

I also have a list of things that I want to accomplish and the target dates for each. This keeps me motivated and moving forward toward all my goals. This is also how I avoid stress and getting wound up. Having a list and marking things off as I complete them lets me know that even if I did not get everything on my list done, I can still feel great about what I accomplished and move forward the next day.

Stress is part of life and cannot be avoided completely, but how you handle stress is what makes a big difference in your life. When you let stress or events get the best of you and get angry or act in a destructive way, it does not make the stress go away. It just magnifies it. Throwing a tantrum or yelling like a child is not only embarrassing, but it is very hard on your body. Your heart starts racing, your blood pressure goes up, and sometimes it is hard to calm yourself down. This leads to feeling out of control and overwhelmed. When you get overwhelmed by anything in your life, it takes control of your emotions and your health. By breaking down everything into bite-size pieces and handling each little part one at a time you will feel more in control and able to handle the rest of the things you need to do. Acting out or getting angry never solves anything and will, in fact, increase your stress.

## YOGA

Yoga is a great way to actively bring about a state of calm and balance to the body. I used to take a yoga class at least two times per week. I did this for stress relief. I was a single parent trying to support my son and myself by running my own business and working as an actor. Yoga gave me fifty minutes to stretch, relax, breathe, and calm my mind. I had already done my morning exercise and started my work day.

Taking a yoga class during the day was hard to fit in, but I found it actually gave me more time in my day because the breathing and stretching helped me to focus on what was important. I turned off my phone and told myself, *whoever calls I can get back to them when I'm finished.* This really made the rest of my day go much smoother and helped me handle whatever came up in a very calm manner.

## MEDITATION

Meditation is another way to relieve stress and focus on what is important. Breathing becomes labored when we get stressed. Meditation helps you to center yourself and clear your mind. Sitting and clearing your mind like this helps you relax, relieves stress, and calms you. Have you noticed how your mind races over a million thoughts at once when you are stressed? It's hard to accomplish anything when you feel like that. Taking time to meditate helps you take a much-needed break from everything and restart again calm and centered.

## GUIDED IMAGERY

Guided imagery is very helpful when trying to reduce stress by focusing on breathing and relaxing images. I listen to a variety of guided imagery CDs when I want to focus my mind, relax, and reduce stress. I also listen to one every night to help me prepare for sleep. If I wake up during the night and cannot go back to sleep, I turn on my guided imagery until I fall asleep.

Guided imagery is also very helpful for reducing stress by talking you through breathing and focusing on positive thoughts. When I have a busy day, trying to unwind can take some time. Listening to guided imagery helps relax me in a matter of minutes every time! Having power over the stress and releasing it makes me feel refreshed and calm after a hard day of work.

There are steps that I follow every night that help me turn off the day and get ready for a relaxing night. Removing clutter and putting my work projects all in one place is great because I can shut my office door and leave my work in the office.

Someone once asked what I did for relaxation. My answer was *sleep*. But she said, "No, sleep is not relaxation. You need to take time to relax." The truth was that I never had time to relax in my entire life. I could not honestly tell her what I did for relaxation because I did not know what that was.

When I met my husband, Jerry, he was a Major in the U.S. Army. He was very happy, very calm, with a great personality and handsome. I never had anyone like this in my life.

The first time we went on a trip together was a three-day weekend. He took trips up to Sea Ranch and rented a house on the beach to take time to relax, and he invited me to come with him. My first question was, "What will we do there?" He said, "Relax." My next question was, "Is there a gym, organic food store, running trails, and what should I bring?" He said, "Just bring yourself and a bathing suit."

The thought of not doing anything and not working for three days was foreign to me. When he picked me up I had a stack of books, weights, exercise bands, running shoes, sandals, and some clothes. He realized then that I did not know how to relax. It was something he needed to teach me.

When we came back from that trip, I felt so refreshed and relaxed I was recharged and ready to go back to work with a whole new attitude and energy I had never had before. I learned just how important it is to take time to relax.

I have a tight schedule every day that starts at 3:00 AM when I get up and go to the gym for a 4:00 AM workout. If I don't get to bed early enough and feel I need more rest, I may sleep an extra half hour, but I am always up and ready to go.

I make a healthy breakfast when I get home and my husband goes to work, then I start on my own work. When I have an appointment, I bring my computer and journals to work on while I am waiting. I don't have much lag time during the day. I break for lunch between 11:30 and 12:00. I make a nutritious lunch and either sit outside or watch a show while I eat, then I head back to work.

I try to stop working at 4:00 PM so I have time to shut down everything before I start preparing dinner. I always make a nutrient dense meal that my husband and I enjoy together. We both finish work before dinner–at least that is the plan. He often gets work calls in the evening and at night. I thought when he retired from the Army we would have a more normal schedule, but that has not happened. We do try to keep on schedule as much as possible while being flexible if something comes up.

On a normal night, we will have a leisurely dinner. It is important to eat slowly and properly chew your food. Gulping down food just causes indigestion and overeating. Then we clean up the kitchen. I set out my gym clothes for the next morning, then brush and floss my teeth, which lets me know eating time is over and it is time to relax. I close the blackout curtains in our bedroom and turn off all the lights. We watch a funny show that I recorded, read a book, stretch, yoga or listen to relaxation CDs, then go to bed.

## SLEEP

Sleep is always very important for your body to be able to rest and repair. It also reduces stress. Lack of sleep can cause a lot of stress and create bad habits like using over-the-counter sleep aids to help you sleep. Prescription medications may be prescribed to help you sleep and to deal with anxiety. Lack of sleep itself can cause anxiety. If you take these medications it may be hard to wake up the next morning and to get your day started. When you have no energy, or have a medication or alcohol hangover, it will cause you to crave caffeine, sugar, and extra food.

After 9/11 Jerry and I knew he would be changing duty station to prepare to go to war. This caused me a great deal of anxiety, and I had insomnia. After a few nights of not sleeping I found it hard to keep my schedule. Then I started worrying about not getting enough sleep. This is not a good thing to do because it makes the mind very active when it should be calming down and getting ready for sleep. I looked for help in the holistic community.

Acupuncture is something I found to be very helpful for calming my nerves and helping me relax, which in turn helps me sleep. In Traditional Chinese Medicine, it is believed that disease is caused by a disruption to the flow of energy, or *qi*, in the body. Tiny needles are gently inserted just below the surface of the skin through specific neurohormonal pathways to stimulate the nerve (https://www.livescience.som/29494-acupuncture.html June 21, 2017). The needles are so tiny they do not cause any pain. While the needles are in place, all you do is rest. When the treatment is completed, the needles are removed. Afterward you feel very relaxed.

## Stress Might Not Be the Problem

There is a time, according to the Mayo clinic, when you should seek medical help. If you are not sure if stress is the cause or if you have taken steps to control your stress, but your symptoms continue, seek help. The doctor may check for potential causes or you might consider seeing a professional counselor or therapist who can help you identify sources of your stress and learn new coping skills.

Seek help immediately if you have chest pain, especially if it occurs during physical activity or is accompanied by shortness of breath, sweating, dizziness, or nausea. Other things to watch for, according to the Mayo Clinic are pain radiating into your shoulder and arm; squeezing or aching sensation in your chest or arms that may spread to your neck, jaw, or back; fatigue; lightshades or sudden dizziness. If you experience any of these symptoms, get emergency help immediately. These may be warning signs of a heart attack and not simply stress (https://www.mayoclinic.org /diseases-conditions/heart-attack/symptoms-causes/ syc-20373106).

My friend was sitting in her living room with her companion and he noticed her rubbing her left arm. When he asked what was wrong she said her arm just hurt a little, but that it was no big deal. Since she was in her nineties and it was her left arm, he took her to the emergency room. She was taken immediately into the operating room because she was having a heart attack. The doctor put a stent in through her arm into her heart to keep the coronary arteries open. She was perfectly fine after that.

It is so much harder for women to detect heart attack symptoms than men. We have to deal with so much pain throughout our lives that we don't think a little in the arm is a big deal. This could have been fatal if she had not been taken into the emergency room right away. I am very thankful that she has such a great friend looking out for her wellbeing.

Heart attack strikes suddenly, but many people have warning signs and symptoms for hours, days, or weeks in advance. The early warning may be recurring chest pain called angina that is triggered by exertion and relieved by rest. Angina is caused by a temporary decrease in blood flow to the heart.

A heart attack differs from a condition in which your heart suddenly stops (sudden cardiac arrest, which occurs when an electrical disturbance disrupts your heart's pumping action and causes blood to stop flowing to the rest of your body). A heart attack can cause cardiac arrest, but it's not the only case. (If you want more information, refer to the Mayo Clinic Healthy Lifestyle website.)

# CHAPTER 15: GETTING ENOUGH SLEEP

Getting enough sleep is one of the most important things that you can do for your body. The body needs time to relax, repair, and rest. Sleep is not something you can make up later. A good night's sleep is necessary for your body to function normally during the day.

When you do not have a good night's sleep, your body does not have the time to repair itself. Lack of sleep can cause memory problems, fatigue, anxiety, depression, and many other issues. Not getting enough sleep may even lead to weight gain because the body is trying to function without enough rest. This creates cravings for sugar, junk foods, and caffeine. Sleep is one of the most important aspects of a healthy lifestyle.

There are different stages of sleep. REM stands for *rapid eye movement*. During this stage, your eyes move quickly. Non-REM (NREM) sleep goes through three stages. In the first stage, the eyes are closed, but it is easy to be wakened. Stage two is light sleep in which the heart rate and body temperature drop. During the third stage the body is in a deep sleep and would be harder to waken. If you were wakened from this stage, you would feel disoriented. It is during NREM sleep that the body repairs, re-grows tissue, builds bones and muscles, and strengthens the immune system. With age, people have less deep sleep and more light sleep.

REM sleep starts about 90 minutes after you fall asleep. The first stage lasts about 10 minutes and each stage gets longer. The last part of REM sleep lasts about an hour. During this stage, your heart rate gets rapid and your breathing quickens. Intense dreams can happen during REM sleep because your brain is more active.

For more information concerning sleep cycles and how they function on average, see https://www.psychologytoday.com/us/blog/between-you-and-me/201307/your-sleep-cycle-revealed.

Melatonin is produced by various tissues of the body although its major source is the pineal gland in the brain. Melatonin is produced naturally from the amino acid, tryptophan, by the pineal gland at night. When the sun goes down and darkness begins, the pineal gland is turned on and begins to activate melatonin. Somewhere around 9:00 p.m. this begins because it is dark outside in most places.

## Prepare for Sleeping

There are ways to create a good sleep atmosphere which will help your body prepare for sleep. Take some time before bed to relax your body by taking a bath, doing light yoga or stretching, or deep breathing. I like to listen to guided relaxation which takes me through deep breathing and guided imagery to help me relax and fall asleep. Meditation is great to do before sleep because it helps you to stop the noise in your head and to relax and become mindful, peaceful, and calm.

Your bedroom should be dark and not have any electronics on or even in the room. If you have a television in your room, cover it up so no light is emitted from it while you are trying to sleep. Cover anything that has a light, no matter how small. These little sources of light can disrupt your sleep. Use a piece of paper or cloth to cover the clock, lights on televisions, and even the light on monitors. If you can move them out of your bedroom altogether, that is best. A sleep mask can block out light and help with sleep, especially when traveling as it is sometimes difficult to cover up all the light sources in your hotel room.

Blackout curtains are great if your room gets evening light from the sun going down, the moon, and streetlights. These curtains can be put behind your regular curtains or you can replace your curtains with ones that are made with blackout material behind them. During the day, curtains can be opened to let in the light, but an hour before bedtime, close them and turn off the lights.

Make sure that everything you need for the night is already in place so you don't have to turn on the lights to find anything. Ear plugs are great if you are in a hotel or noisy neighborhood or if your partner snores. If you have small children ear plugs may not be the best idea.

The temperature of your room is important for a good night's sleep. If the room is too cold, it can wake you up, and if they room is too warm, it can make it hard to fall asleep. Set your thermostat to 63 degrees, which is the ideal temperature for sleeping.

When traveling, ask for a lightweight blanket for the room. Many hotels have heavy comforters on the beds, even during the summer. Having a lightweight blanket will help reduce body temperature. Some hotels have motion detectors on the air conditioner so it turns off at night. Having a lightweight blanket can help you sleep comfortably if the air conditioner shuts off in the middle of the night.

Electronics of any kind should be turned off at least one hour before bed. When you are using a screen, it stimulates the brain and keeps it active. Some people will even say they are addicted to their electronics. Power them down an hour before bedtime! You can read an actual book if you need something to do. Make sure it is something relaxing and not stimulating or something that will give you nightmares. Audio tapes recorded on a small iPod will be the only thing that you can listen to in bed, and it needs to only have sleep guided imagery or relaxing music. I do not recommend putting these on your phone if you listen to them in bed. Having the phone ring or give text alerts will disrupt your sleep. There are sleep machines which provide white noise and help with sleep, too.

After eating dinner, clean and de-clutter your kitchen. Make lunches for the next day, set out what you need for the morning, and prepare the kids for sleep. Brush your teeth, floss, wash your face, and do anything else that requires light. Once you have finished, darken the bedroom and set everything up for a healthy night's sleep.

Starting something before bed interferes with your body's natural sleep cycle. Let your body calm down and get into bed feeling ready for sleep. Cover your eyes if there is a lot of light outside. The darker the room, the better you will sleep.

When my granddaughters are staying with me, I give them each a small flashlight that is bright. I also have a nightlight in the hall and one in the bathroom by their room. I even do this when we are in a hotel. It makes them feel safe and they can find the bathroom if they need to get up at night. I wake easily if I hear them get up and I attend to them and walk them back to bed. I use a flashlight by my bed if I am in a room at someone's house that I am not familiar with or if I am in a hotel. That way, I can find the bathroom without turning on the light.

One thing that disrupts the preparation for sleep is exercising in the evening or close to bedtime. If that is the only time you can exercise, then also do something relaxing close to bedtime like reading a book, taking a warm bath, sitting in a Jacuzzi or steam room, or take a yoga class. Meditation and deep breathing always help relax the mind and the body.

Tryptophan is an amino acid that is found in turkey, dairy products, and supplements. Eating something that contains tryptophan or taking it as a supplement can help with sleep. Consult your doctor if you have sleep problems that last more than a week or two. Ask them about supplements and over the counter sleep aids before taking them.

I have found that eating some turkey always works great, but remember to not use anything with sugar or spices on it. Cottage cheese, yogurt, milk, almonds, garbanzo beans, oats, and eggs also contain tryptophan. Eating a small bowl of cottage cheese or drinking some warm milk helps with sleep.

Eating your dinner a few hours before bed is great because your body has time to digest the food. Eating a large meal right before bed may disrupt your sleep. Food eaten close to bed time is more likely to be stored as fat. During the day, your body burns more calories because you are more active. At night when your body is resting and repairing, it does not need as many calories. Avoid caffeine in the afternoon and evening as well as tobacco and alcohol. They all can disrupt your sleep patterns.

Schedule a regular time to go to bed and to get up in the morning and condition your body so you wake up at the same time every day. Waking up without an alarm is great. By going to bed and getting up at the same time, your body will make this a natural habit. Avoid watching television, eating, and reading in bed. Try not to nap during the day. If you do take a nap, try not to sleep longer than thirty minutes. This is enough time to refresh your body and mind without disrupting your sleep at night. Don't nap in the afternoon or near bedtime. Avoid rigorous exercise three hours before bedtime.

## IF SOMETHING SEEMS WRONG

There are some things that may indicate a serious problem and should be reported to your doctor. Snoring can be a sign of a serious problem. Sleep apnea is a sleep disorder that disrupts normal sleep patterns and can be very dangerous. Sleep disorders can be diagnosed through doing a sleep study. People with sleep apnea can stop breathing during the night and have disrupted sleep patterns.

Narcolepsy is a disorder which causes one to fall asleep while doing normal activities during the day. It is an inability to stay awake. This is a very dangerous condition that can be diagnosed by a doctor. Falling asleep every time you sit down and rest for a few minutes is not healthy. If you have any condition that is not normal or if you are snoring, gasping for air, or waking often during the night consult your doctor.

# CHAPTER 16: FITTING EXERCISE INTO YOUR DAILY ROUTINE

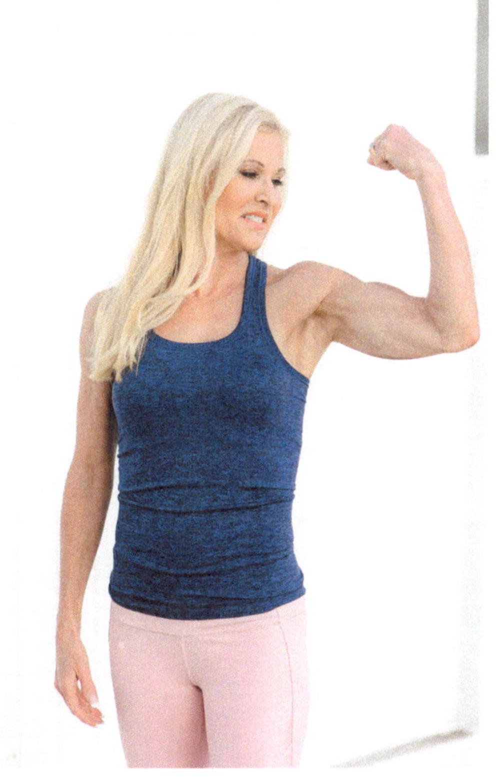

### EXERCISE DAILY

Have you ever seen people who are in great shape and wish you could look like them? Do you see people who eat healthy and wish you had the will power to do the same? Do you ever see an athlete and think it would be great to be able to do what they can do?

I can tell you from personal experience that you can achieve whatever you believe you can. What would you try if you knew you would not fail? This is a great question to ask yourself and write down everything that you come up with as soon as it pops into your mind. It is a great way to get into the frame of mind to be successful. All the things that you know you can achieve you will achieve. The first step is to know that you set your mind up to achieve.

Your brain is a very complicated machine and it is also very simplistic in its desires and needs. The brain requires protein to build neurotransmitters called message transmitters that help brain cells communicate. The brain needs carbohydrates from whole foods such as legumes, beans, fruits, and vegetables for high-quality fuel in order to function. The carbohydrates are broken down into glucose to be used by the brain cell activity. The brain also needs water to stay properly hydrated and working efficiently. And it also needs stimulation from the outside world as well as from the inside world.

Have you ever heard of a *weekend warrior*? This is someone who only works out on the weekends. Some people do extremely hard workouts on the weekend and light workouts during the week. Some people only workout on the weekend. If you are not doing any exercise at all this is a good time for you to start. It does not matter what type of exercise you start with as long as you start doing some form of exercise. Making exercise part of your daily routine will make you feel great!

## POSITIVE ATTRACTION

Besides eating whole foods and having a healthy eating plan, you also need to have positive influence around you. We talked about this earlier, but it is worth mentioning again. It is vital to your success. If you believe that you will be successful at whatever you want to do, you are much closer to achieving your goals. Many books—the Bible, *As a Man Thinketh*by James Allen, and *The Power of Positive Thinking* by Norman Vincent Peale teach this truth. Buddha taught that, *what you think you become.* All of these people and many different cultures all teach the same thing, which is the power of thinking you are what you want to become. Act as if you already have what you want. Talk to yourself as though you already are the person you want to be. This is very powerful and will help bring your goals into reality.

If you constantly tell yourself that you are a failure, that you cannot eat healthy, that you cannot lose weight, you hate to exercise, that you cannot get up early, or you don't have time to eat healthy or exercise, you plant seeds of doubt and failure in your mind. Changing the way you communicate with yourself is a very powerful way of becoming the person you want to be. Loving yourself will make you more loveable and attractive to others. It will make you more powerful and attract people who are like-minded.

You don't want to attract negative people who are always down on themselves and others. You want strong powerful people who are the "movers and shakers" of the world to be around you. What are groups of people who have the same goal in mind? They are supportive, positive, and will help you focus on your goal. People who have the same goals in mind, whether it is starting a healthy eating plan, being a more positive person, or starting an exercise program, are the people you want to surround yourself with. These are the people who will be supportive in your new life style. If you are already doing these things they will be a support system for you to continue moving forward in a positive way and achieving great things. Being around like-minded positive people really helps bring about a positive way of thinking that can lead to your goals being realized. When you put yourself in the state of mind to be successful, you will be successful. Making health your top priority and knowing that you will succeed at being healthy is what will help you achieve those goals.

## If You're New to Exercising

*For those who have never done any exercise or who have any physical limitations or health issues, check with your doctor before starting any new exercise program.*

It is always best to start slow instead of jumping into a rigorous workout. The gym has a variety of exercise options available to you. If you have never gone to a gym before, ask someone to show you how to use the machines or weights. Most gyms will give you a free tour and help get you started well. There are many amenities that come with a gym membership. There are many classes, cardio machines, free weights, and weight machines. There are also showers, dressing rooms, saunas, Jacuzzis, and massage therapists. Memberships are very low in cost considering all that you can get out of them.

Joining a gym is a great way to get the proper training you need. A professional trainer can teach you proper technique for lifting weights. Proper form is very important regardless of the type of exercise you do. Your trainer can help you achieve your goals.

And just in case any of you ladies don't know, you can stop worrying about something right now. If you start lifting weights will your muscles develop like a man's do? The answer is no! Women do not have enough testosterone (male hormone) to make their muscles big like a man's. Some women have more testosterone than others, but they still will not develop like a man.

It is important to lift weights to keep your muscles strong so they can support your body. More muscle means more calories are being burned. The more muscle you have, the easier it is to lose weight. When you gain muscle, you will look and feel better.

Your weight may go up on the scale, but as long as you are gaining muscle, not fat, it is fine. You can develop great muscles and look great. You will also be able to eat more without getting fat if you exercise, doing cardiovascular and weight training. The freedom you feel from being physically fit is like none other.

The gym is great for beginners and you can go at your own pace. It is important not to try to keep up with others in the class who might be more advanced than you. It will become obvious which people are more experienced, but don't let that bother you. Each person in the gym or in your class has been at the exact place you are now as a beginner. Showing up at the gym is a great accomplishment. Some people are more coordinated than others, some are stronger, but everyone is there for the same reason, and that is to get a great workout. As you get comfortable with lifting weights or taking classes, you will get stronger and more coordinated.

Starting a walking program is a very simple way to work into an exercise program. Walking can be done through your neighborhood, at a track, or on a treadmill at home or at the gym. A brisk walk can get your blood circulating and may be the perfect place to start if you have not done any type of exercise.

If you have already started a brisk walking program you can start a walk-run. This is just what it sounds like. Walk for a few minutes and then run for whatever period of time you are able. It does not have to be a fast run. It can be a little jog. This is a way of conditioning the body for more vigorous exercise.

I have known many people who have dropped a lot of excess weight by just walking. One of them in particular was scheduled to have knee surgery. The fear of surgery got her up and walking every day to lose the excess weight she was carrying. Every day she walked a little farther and a little faster. She lost over 100 pounds and was walking at a very fast pace. Her knee stopped hurting and she never had to have the surgery. The extra weight she was carrying was putting stress on her knee. By losing weight and getting stronger, she was able to avoid the surgery.

## EXERCISE ONE HOUR EACH DAY

One thing that is the same for everyone is the amount of time we all have in a day. There are 24 hours in your day and it is up to you to use them wisely. Schedule an hour per day for exercise and choose something that is of interest to you or that you can do for an hour.

Everyone works, from the stay-at-home mom or dad to the high-paid executive or business owner. We all have a job to do every single day of the week. Even on weekends we are either working or busy with shopping, errands, kids' events, sports, and a variety of chores.

If you start your day early and go to the gym before work, it is easier to get your exercise done every day without interruptions. Going to the gym between 4:00 and 6:00 a.m.gets your workout done early, energizing you to go start your day. By planning your meals in advance and packing a lunch and breakfast, you go straight to work after your workout. You have healthy meals ready and you've started your day in a very healthy way.

When you first begin exercising daily, it may be difficult to start out with a full hour of exercise. Don't let that stop you. The duration may not be a full hour, but that is something to strive for. The hour can be thirty minutes of cardiovascular exercise and thirty minutes of weight training. Any exercise that gets your heart rate up is cardiovascular in nature. This includes things like jumping rope, rowing, elliptical training, stair-stepper, treadmill, hiking, biking, and aerobic classes. Dancing is also a great exercise and is something you can do in a class or at home.

Take your time to find something you can stick with or try something that you have always wanted to try. Making a conscious decision to exercise is the most important think you can do along with eating healthy. It does not matter how many things you try as long as you keep exercising in some way. It helps to enjoy what you are doing, but it is not mandatory. There may be an exercise that you don't love, but you do it every day to get your exercise. Exercise may be hard at first, but it will become easier in time.

Some people may think they are not morning people, but I have helped many people become morning people just by talking about how to plan their day around morning exercise. Once they started getting up early and going to the gym or going for a walk or a run, they found it is the most peaceful time of day to take care of themselves.

Get everything ready the night before. Set out your exercise clothes for the morning and have your snack to eat before you leave. If everything is ready to go when you wake up, it makes everything easier for you to get up and exercise in the morning.

If you have little ones at home set up a home gym and take that time to exercise before the kids get up. Buy a spinning bike, dumbbells, and a stability ball. Be sure to keep your equipment out of the reach of young children as they could get hurt trying to use your equipment when you're not there. If you are a couple with children, one of you can exercise while the other watches the kids and alternate days or times of day. Do whatever you must do in order to get some exercise into your life. Where there is a will there is a way. Just keep in mind that this is part of your healthy lifestyle.

I put my weights away in the closet and my spinning bikes in the sunroom. When I am ready to exercise, I bring them to an open area of my house so I have enough room to do all my exercise. My newest piece of equipment is a Pilates Studio Reformer with a tower to convert into a Pilates Cadillac. There are hundreds of exercises that can be done with this piece of equipment and they all focus on strengthening core muscles. I have learned many different movements with my Pilates instructor and I can practice them at home on my Reformer.

## TRY NEW THINGS

Trying new things is always fun. Be curious about exercise. Pretend that you are a kid who gets a new toy or a bicycle. Exercise is not a chore. It is fun!

When I left southern California and the beach, I felt lost because the beach was where I always went to exercise. I started to skate and ride a bike on the trail of San Jose and Los Gatos, California, and I loved it. The weather is colder in northern California, so I had to figure out how to get outside in the cold weather and how to dress for it. I am a true southern California girl who was used to the beach and warm weather all year long. It was hard for me to get used to the northern climate until I found the right clothes. I joined a gym so I could exercise inside when the weather was rainy or cold.

I started running after I was diagnosed with colon cancer in 1994. I did not think I could get used to the changes. I met a friend at the park who told me about an upcoming race. I told her I was not a runner and could not run in a race. She told me I had three months to train.

The race was the Dammit Race in Los Gatos, California. She showed me the trail where the race took place. I started running the next day. I had been doing aerobics and step aerobics classes at the gym and lifting light weights, so I thought I would be able to run the entire way. There were three steep hills and a very steep, rocky downhill on the other side of the dam. I had to talk the hills, and I wasn't able to run the whole distance.

I did enjoy being out in nature and getting fresh air and sunshine. I set my goal to run in the race, and I went to the trail and did my practice run whenever I could. It took me a few weeks to make it all the way without stopping, but I finally made it. Every time I got to the end of the trail, I felt great! I kept telling myself that I could do it, and finally I was able to complete it. I used the same determination to get through a colon resection and beat colon cancer to get to the top of the hills and to run the entire loop through the hills.

Be determined to make your exercise a joyful experience. Give it an important place in your life because it can save your life. Think of a time when you achieved something great. Recreate the feeling in your mind. Visualize yourself enjoying every minute of your exercise program. If you are training for a race or some type of competition, visualize yourself finishing strong. Visualize yourself being successful and you will succeed. This is a very powerful way of training your mind as well as your body. Take that feeling and apply it to whatever type of exercise you are doing. Use your inner strength and positive feelings to help you try new things and to find exercise that you love.

There are many ways to increase your activity level throughout the day. Use the stairs instead of the elevator. Park your car at the end of the parking lot instead of near the store. Walk to the park or to school or ride your bike. I loved living in Campbell, California, because I could ride my bike on the trail that was just a mile from my house. I would get on the trail and take it all the way to the Los Gatos Creek Trail, up the face of Lexington Dam. There was a road that went all the way around the dam and through the trees in a loop, then I would ride back home. It was about a 2 ½ hour ride and it was beautiful. That was something I looked forward to on the weekends.

## Drop Your Excuses

When we moved to Fort Hood Texas we joined a gym near our home. The entire cardio room was dark. I could not even see how to start the machine. When I asked the person at the front desk why the room was dark, she told me that women do not like anyone to see them work out.

Do not worry about what other people may be thinking of you because everyone had to start somewhere. Everyone that shows up at the gym or does any type of exercise should be proud of themselves for taking the time to exercise. No one is perfect and the only thing people will see when you start going to the gym or starting any type of exercise is that you are putting in the time and effort to improve your health.

If you go to any gym, track, or running trail, you will see a variety of body shapes, sizes, ages, and genders and they are all there to improve their health. When you think about going to a gym or track, all you have to worry about is getting there early enough to get a parking spot. Once you are there, you are unstoppable. You are on the way to getting the body you want and to living a healthy lifestyle.

This is a great time to use your positive self-talk. Tell yourself that you are amazing, positive, have a strong body and can get through your exercise routine. The only thing holding you back from getting what you want is the excuses you tell yourself. Don't make any excuses. Take action today by starting an exercise program and motivate yourself to achieve optimal health. Whatever you do to move your body is a great start to achieving your goals.

The benefits of exercise are many, starting with making you feel great about yourself. People have experienced great joy exercising along with losing weight, lowering blood pressure and cholesterol, and managing blood sugar. What exercise does for your mind and body will amaze you. Don't let insecurities keep you from exercising. There is great joy and fulfillment waiting for you!

Watching your body change into a strong, lean physique is something that will make you very proud of yourself. Being fit and strong will improve your self-esteem and help you do things that used to tire you out like walking up a flight of stairs or playing with your kids. You will be amazed by what you can achieve when you are physically fit.

## EXERCISE ALONE OR WITH A WORKOUT BUDDY

The great thing about working out alone is that you are on your own schedule. You don't have to wait for anyone and you can do whatever you want to do. When I started exercising I always did it alone. I would go skating on the strand at the beach in southern California and go body surfing and swimming. When I first started going to the gym I went by myself, took step aerobics classes, and had a trainer show me how to lift weights. On the weekends, I would ride my bike through the hills of Los Gatos, California, by myself. Being alone gave me time to reflect and be thankful to be alive and able to do the things I was doing.

If exercising alone isn't appealing to you, there are usually other people out riding their bikes or running on the trails and there are always people at the gym. Go wherever you want to exercise and find someone who is working out in the gym or riding at a fast past on the trail, then try to keep up with them. You will end up meeting new friends, and if you want a workout partner, they are not hard to find.

There are like-minded people everywhere that are trying to improve their health by exercising. Introduce yourself and ask if they would like to work out with you. People who work out are usually friendly and very approachable. It will be very easy to make new friends and have someone to work out with if you ask.

## TAKING CARE OF INJURIES

It is hard to take time off when you are used to working out every day, but there are times when it is necessary. If you get injured, it is important to seek medical attention. If your doctor gives you permission to walk or to lift weights, then you can continue with a modified workout until you heal. If the doctor wants you to rest, it is best to follow that order and rest. It does not do any good to try to work out through an injury.

As you know, I like to use a heart rate monitor when I exercise all the time, even if I am just walking. There have been times when I had an injury or reason I could not do my regular exercise routine. But I was able to walk and track my exercise by wearing the monitor. Normally I burn between 450-525 calories during an hour of cardiovascular exercise. Walking, I would maybe burn 150-200 calories in an hour. It was important for me to stick to my healthy eating plan and to walk three times a day. In the beginning I could only walk about 20 minutes at a time. As I was feeling better, I increased the duration, but if I felt any pain I would have to rest.

When I was a runner, I injured my Achilles' tendon. I wanted to keep running, but it was too painful. I went to the trail in the hills nearby and started walking and stretching. I found another runner doing the same thing, so we recovered together. It was not long before we were back to running, and I made a new friend in the process.

Letting your body heal and repair is one of the most important things to do with an injury. To rest, ice and elevate your injury. Seek the help of a trained professional chiropractor, physical therapist, massage therapist or acupuncturist. If you need to see a doctor and he tells you a surgery is needed, be sure to get several other opinions before going under the knife. I know sometimes it may be necessary, but be sure you are making the right decision. Choose physical therapy and other therapies prior to surgery. Surgery may be a last resort. If you do need surgery for any reason, ask before the surgery if you will be able to walk during your recovery. Depending on the type of surgery and the area involved, it may be fine to walk or to lift light weights. By following the doctor's instructions during recovery you will get back to exercise sooner than if you try to return too soon and reinjure yourself. Be sure that your doctor clears you for exercise, even if you are just going to walk.

## MIX IT UP

Exercise keeps you feeling healthy, young, and fit. It is not just about how you look. It is also about how you feel. Exercise brings great joy to your life because it increases blood flow throughout the body. Cardiovascular exercise will get your heart pumping, help to keep your heart strong, and burn a lot of calories. Lifting weights will build muscles which will increase your strength and increase your metabolism. Doing a combination of cardiovascular exercise and weight training is a winning combination.

This does not mean you must go to the gym every day. Take the weekend to go running, biking, hiking, or swimming. One of the many advantages of daily exercise is that it keeps you feeling and looking young. At the same time, you will be able to do more of the things in life that healthy people do, like running in a race and playing with your children and grandchildren. Exercise IS fun! Getting up early in the morning and going to the gym or going on a run, bike ride, or brisk walk is the best way to start the day. Make it a point to do some form of exercise every day.

There are so many types of exercise it will be easy to find a program you can stick to and enjoy. Exercise is not a chore; it is a gift. Good health is a gift you can give yourself and your family. It is great to exercise with a friend or significant other, but it is also something you can do alone.

Fit exercise into your daily routine and get your kids involved. Take a family bike ride, play or run at the park, play basketball, tennis or racquetball. There are so many ways to get exercise and have fun doing it. Many people are using Fit Bits or some type of step counter to motivate them to move their bodies. Knowing you are improving your health should be a great motivator.

# CHAPTER 17: TRACY'S EXERCISE ROUTINE

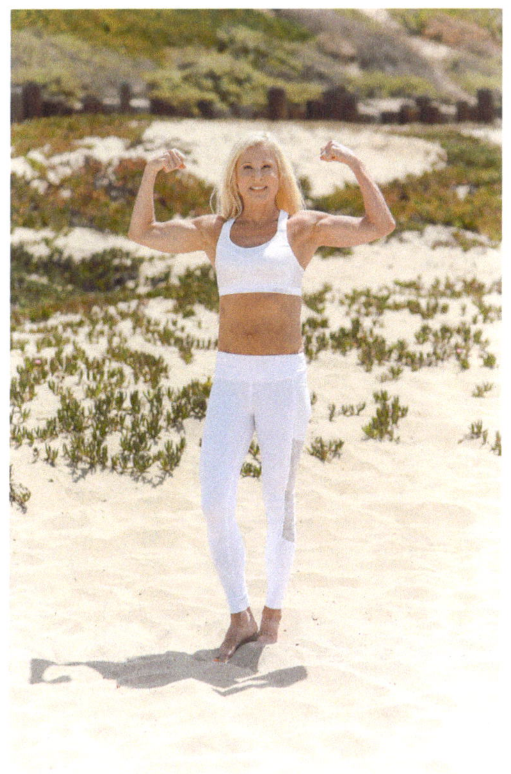

## TRACY'S DAILY EXERCISE

During the week, I go to the gym early in the morning. It is a great time to work out. It does not interfere with the rest of my day. There is not much happening at 4:00 am to interfere with my workout. Even though there are other people at the gym it is not as crowded in the morning as it is in the afternoon and evenings. My gym is open 24 hours a day which is great because some gyms don't open until 5 or 6 am which doesn't fit well with my schedule.

I usually use the elliptical trainer or stationary bike first then go lift weights. There are times when I feel like just lifting weights or just doing cardiovascular exercise, like the elliptical or the bike.

I have two spinning bikes at home. My husband and I ride them if we have early appointments or don't have time to get to the gym. This is a great piece of equipment to have in your home. I can burn 500 calories while watching *Dancing with the Stars* (DWTS) or listening to music. I find music to be a great motivator. Choosing fast-paced music keeps me spinning at a good fast pace. I also love the music and the dancing on *DWTS*. It keeps me motivated and I burn a lot of calories. Jerry and I ride our spinning bikes on the weekend and then go to the gym to lift weights.

My heart rate monitor also serves as a great motivator for me. I can do interval training where I pedal really fast for a minute or two and then slow down for a minute or two. Alternating speeds, adjusting the tension to make it harder to pedal and standing up to pedal are ways to vary the workout on a spinning bike. It's so fun and it never gets boring.

I can check my monitor to see how high my heart rate is and make sure I am working hard enough. This can also be determined by my breathing. You should be able to talk while you are doing cardiovascular exercise as opposed to being out of breath. This is a good way to make sure you aren't over-exerting yourself.

I have been doing this form of exercise for many years, so I know what my heart rate should be. However, when starting an exercise program, be sure you to check with your doctor.

People have asked me how many years it takes to get into shape. I ask them what kind of shape they are talking about. Getting into shape means different things to different people. The main thing is that being healthy must be the top priority.

If you are eating a healthy meal plan and following an exercise routine, everything else will fall into place. If your goal is to improve your health, this is a great plan for you to follow. If you are trying to lose weight, it is also a great plan for you. Eating a healthy meal plan will also help to keep your blood sugar from spiking or dropping too low and help to lower cholesterol. Do not stop taking medication without talking with your doctor.

When you do cardiovascular exercise, you burn a lot of calories, improve blood flow, and the condition of your heart. Lifting weights helps build muscle which burns calories all day long. This is a positive reason for lifting weights. Muscle gets lost during the aging process. If you don't keep your muscles strong, your metabolism will slow down.

The number of calories burned during exercise gives you an idea of how many calories you can eat. Whether you are trying to lose weight, maintain weight, gain muscle, or improve your health, knowing how many calories you need to consume is important. If you eat too many calories, you will gain weight. If you eat too few, your metabolism slows down.

This doesn't mean that you have to count calories. I have done all the hard work for you. All you need to do is follow my healthy eating plan and add some form of exercise. If you buy something in a package, just be sure to read the label to determine whether or not it is a healthy choice.

An average woman may need 2000 calories a day to maintain weight and 1500 to lose one pound per week. An average man needs 2500 calories to maintain weight and about 2000 to lose one pound a week. The amount differs depending on your fitness level, the amount of muscle you have, what you eat, and the type of exercise you are doing. If you are trying to lose weight, you should eat at least the minimum number of calories per day in the form of lean protein, healthy complex carbohydrates, and healthy fats. Eating healthy meals and snacks and doing daily exercise will help you achieve your goals.

## When to Modify Your Exercise

Modify your exercise if you are not feeling well or if you are tired. If you are feeling exhausted or sick, take the day off from exercising. You can go for a walk or do a yoga DVD at home. Don't push yourself when you are sick. One or two days off from the gym will not hurt you. Exercising when you are sick may actually hurt you.

There may be days when you just feel bored with your exercise routine or need a change of pace. Try taking a class at the gym or go on a run or a walk with a friend. Make plans to meet with a friend or go out to lunch after your workout. Sometimes you just need a little variation to your exercise or daily routine to put life back into your exercise program.

## GET INVOLVED WITH TEAM SPORTS

Finding something you like to do may involve joining a team sport or any group activity. As long as you are moving your body and getting some exercise, it's a great day. There are many team sports like volley ball, baseball, tennis, racquetball, football, gymnastics, cheerleading, and dance classes. If you get motivated by joining team sports, then find a team or even a running or walking group. There are many options available at the gym or the local community center. Community announcements are posted, many of them online, and they are free or very low cost.

I used to take tap dancing when I was very little. My mom took me out when I was five, but I always loved it. I joined an adult tap class at the community center, and it was great! I was the youngest one in the class. I could not keep up with the ladies who were 20 years older than I was. They were great dancers and had so much energy. I went to the class after work every Tuesday and Thursday nights for two hours. We learned two dance numbers and performed at a dance recital at the park with all the other dancers from other classes.

## JUST DO SOMETHING!

Not knowing what to do or where to start can sometimes stop people from doing things. Just go out and do something. It does not matter what it is as long as you are moving your body and having fun.

Some people will say the best part of working out is when they are finished. But they really love it or they wouldn't be there. Don't let the fear of being different or not being as fit as someone else stop you from joining in.

Think of yourself as an athlete whether you are one or not. Think of every day as your training for the main event called life. Every workout, every meal, everything you do is leading up to the main event. Don't forget the little short training races that you have to run before the marathon or the Iron Man Triathlon (swimming and biking followed by a marathon).

Life throws all sorts of curve balls your way, and you don't know what is ahead of you, no matter how much you plan or how hard you try. But know that if you are physically fit and using my healthy eating plan, you will be better equipped to handle whatever life brings your way.

It is said that God does not give you more than you can handle. It is also said that what does not kill you makes you stronger. If you are prepared for the curve ball and you train for the main event called life, you will succeed and get through whatever comes your way.

I know that what I have been dealt in my own life has been physically and emotionally overwhelming. Not one person should go through what I have been through, but I know that it has made me stronger and wiser. I know that I can stand up to anything because I have survived in my life.

Exercise is a very important part of my life and it should be a very important part of your life also. Think of it as your morning cup of coffee or shot of adrenalin. It gets you up and moving. It gets your blood flowing and makes you feel great. Exercise is better than any coffee or pastry in the world. It can be incorporated into your healthy eating plan to make you feel good and strong.

When you are around people who are working out and eating healthy, it makes you want to do the same, especially if they look and feel great. It is infectious. You see people biking, running, and lifting weights at the gym and it motivates you to get involved, too.

Find the people who are really working out hard, who look like they are enjoying their exercise, and imitate them. This is really important for people who have never worked out before or who are having trouble getting started. Everyone has to start somewhere. No one wakes up looking great and strong; they have to work at it.

## FIND YOUR APPROACH TO EXERCISE

Different ways of approaching exercise and finding what you really love are important for keeping you on a daily exercise routine. You can take one day off a week if you are training hard and eating right. If you do moderate exercise and have no injuries, it is okay to work out every day.

Take time to stretch and to warm up. Try taking yoga class. Yoga helps with flexibility, strength, stability, and it calms the mind. It also teaches you to breathe, which is so important for your body. Yoga connects mind, body, and soul. It gets you in touch with your body and your breathing, and it helps you to relax into the poses.

Do not try to push yourself beyond your limits or over-stretch. If you are taking yoga for the first time, ask your instructor to help you with modified poses. Talking with the instructor prior to the class and letting him/her know that you are new to yoga or are returning from an injury is good. It gives them insight into what modifications you may need. If your instructor does not offer modifications, then find another class. The job of an instructor is to instruct and give modifications for those who are new or not as limber or strong as other people may be.

I had this experience with a yoga instructor who had many people who came to her class all the time. She worked at their level which was very advanced. The class was not posted as an advanced yoga class. She did not give any modified instruction for new people or those who could not do advanced moves or stretches.

I spoke with her before the class and asked her to make modifications if I needed them. You can get seriously injured in yoga if you over-stretch or if you try to force your body into a pose. This instructor did not give me any modifications, so I had to do simpler poses that I knew I could do when she was giving an advanced move. For a class offered through a low-end gym, it was very advanced. She did not like me doing different poses, but I did not want to hurt myself or waste my time by leaving her class.

This is not how an instructor should be. Even in cycling classes, the instructor gives cues for people who cannot keep up or who need a slower, easier pace. Be sure to speak up if this happens to you. For the most part, instructors are very nice and willing to help newcomers. Most of them will ask at the beginning of the class if there are any people new to the class they are teaching. This will make your class more enjoyable for you and for the instructor, too.

Classes like cycling or body pump may look intimidating to someone who has never taken one of these classes before. Don't let this keep you from attending a class and giving it your all. You are not in competition with anyone but yourself. By this I mean, challenge yourself to do a little more or do a little better each time.

When you attend a class for the first time, show up 10 minutes early and speak with the instructor and let them know you are new and might need some modified help until you can catch up with the rest of the class.

Remember that you may not be able to reach the level of some people in the class. There will always be people that have been taking the class for years or they may have natural ability, flexibility or be stronger than other people. This is something that you know going into the class so you don't overwork, over-train, or over-stretch.

A good instructor will walk around or at least look at everyone's form. Keep this in mind with any type of class or group participation activity. Don't miss out on a chance to try something new just because others are more advanced than you are.

There are many ways to fit exercise into your day. Take time before work or at lunch, or both, to get some exercise. Go to the gym in the morning and go for a walk or a run at lunch. Skip lunch and go to the gym. Eat lunch when you finish your workout. There are so many benefits to exercising. It is never too late to start an exercise program.

## A Word about Pilates

Pilates is one of the greatest forms of exercise I have found to keep my body strong and maintain my health. Pilates focuses on maintaining core strength and breathing. It is very important to maintain core strength in order to support your whole body.

I have a great Pilates instructor I work with in Hermosa Beach, California. I started working with her after I had a major surgery. I was not getting better in physical therapy and I wanted to use Pilates for my rehabilitation. I was seeing a physical therapist when I started working with her.

After a few sessions, it became clear to me that she was helping me more than the therapist was. I started seeing her two times a week for the month I was in California. I have been working with her ever since.

I really feel my small muscles and core muscles working when I do Pilates. My family still lives in California. I love to go back to the beach and visit my friends and do my Pilates with my great instructor. I go to the gym in the morning take a walk or a bike ride at the beach in the afternoon. This makes me feel better than anything else.

Pilates is such a great form of exercise and core strengthening that I bought a professional Reformer for my home that also converts into a Cadillac. That means I can do the exercises of two pieces of equipment with one Reformer. This enables me to continue with all the exercises I learn with my instructor after I return home each time. And I can learn more exercises to do as well.

I go to California every few months to work out with my instructor and learn more exercises to do on my Reformer at home. It is essential to find an instructor who pays close attention to make sure you are using correct form and getting the core muscles to fire.

I went to several instructors before I found the right one. Pilates instructors vary in training and experience. Find one who has been properly trained and can give you positions and exercises that are right for you. Intuition is very important, too.

There are hundreds of movements and positions that can be done on a Reformer and on a Cadillac Reformer. Joseph Pilates invented the first Reformer as a way to treat and rehabilitate soldiers that were injured during World War I. The success was so great that it has been around since that time and has become more popular throughout the years.

## EATING WHEN YOU CAN'T WORK OUT

There will be some times when you are unable to work out. The most important thing to do at those times is to maintain my healthy eating plan.

If you have to take time off of working out for any reason, pay close attention to what you are eating. You won't need to eat as many calories as you do when you are running or working out hard. Cut out some of the extra calories by eating smaller portions during that time. Do not diet because your body still needs calories to maintain muscle and to repair.

Stay away from all the junk and empty calorie foods and concentrate on your organic fruits and vegetables and lean protein. Eating these healthy choices provides your body with the nutrients, vitamins, minerals, fiber, etc., it needs to get and stay healthy. By doing this you maintain your fitness and keep your weight in check.

It is wise to not drink alcohol while you are in recovery from an injury or when you are taking medication. Alcohol causes you to gain weight very rapidly due to extra calories and it slows your metabolism.

When your body is trying to heal, it is also important to give it the nutrients it needs. Staying on my healthy eating plan, even if you have stop exercise while you heal, will ensure that you are giving your body what it needs in order to recover.

## FINAL THOUGHTS

The goal is to keep up with your exercise no matter where you are or what is going on. It is important to take at least that one hour a day to do some form of exercise. Move your body and get your heart pumping and your blood flowing. There are so many people who are living into their 90s now, and the ones who are in the best shape both mentally and physically are the ones who get daily exercise and eat a healthy diet. They take time to enjoy life and have fun and friendship. Many people are still working in their 90s, doing things that use the brain and keep them on their toes.

My father-in-law is a very good example of this. He was doing his own taxes, investing in the stock market, and helping his kids make wise investment decisions. He continued stock investing, reading the papers, watching news programs, and always learning new things. He was always very positive and optimistic until his very last day on earth. He would always tell me to take time to sit down and put my feet up and always have fun and take good care of myself and of my husband.

Life is what you make of it and how you spend every day. Choosing to be happy and healthy is one of the best decisions you will ever make. Don't waste time on anything negative and don't sit around feeling sorry for yourself or making excuses for not doing things that you want to do. Find a way to accomplish all your goals and live life to the fullest. Remember, this is not a dress rehearsal. This is your life. You need to take full control and full advantage of every opportunity to enjoy each day and make the most out of every hour in every day.

# CHAPTER 18: RECIPES

### TRACY'S VEGGIE SCRAMBLE

- 3-6 egg whites
- 2 egg yolks
- Zucchini, chopped
- Bell pepper, chopped
- Mushrooms, chopped
- Broccoli, chopped

Place chopped vegetables in a non-stick frying pan and cook over medium heat until desired tenderness is reached. Whip eggs and add to vegetables. Cook until eggs are fully cooked. Makes 1-2 servings.

### TRACY'S FRENCH TOAST

- 4 egg whites
- 1 whole egg
- 2 slices Ezekiel raisin bread
- Stevia
- Cinnamon
- Agave or pure maple syrup

Whip together the egg whites and whole eggs in a bowl. Dip each slice of bread into the egg mixture, coating well on both sides. Then place dipped bread slices into non-stick frying pan. Sprinkle a light dusting of stevia and cinnamon on each slice. Cook on both sides until they reach desired firmness. Serve hot. May add a drizzle of agave or pure maple syrup.

## Tracy's Eggs Benedict

- 1 whole egg
- 1 slice Ezekiel sesame bread or Ezekiel English muffin, toasted
- Thick-sliced (at 2.5), oven-roasted turkey breast (nitrate-, hormone-, and antibiotic-free)
- Heart Smart or Veggie cheese
- Spinach & tomato (optional)

Poach egg (if making more than 1 serving, use 1 egg per slice of toast) in medium boiling water with a pinch of salt added. Poaching will take 2-3 minutes. While egg is poaching, toast the bread and heat the oven-roasted turkey in a frying pan on low heat.

Place turkey on top of the toast, then top with poached egg. Add Heart Smart or veggie cheese on top, and heat for 10 seconds in microwave. Add spinach and tomato to give it a new twist, if you like.

## Breakfast Burrito

Cook scrambled egg whites or whites with one yolk. Heat organic vegetarian refried beans. Heat a large Ezekiel or Alvarado Street tortilla shell. Put beans and egg on tortilla and add salsa and a tablespoon of low-fat cottage cheese.

## Tofu Scramble

Heat steamed vegetables or chop onion, bell pepper, mushrooms, and firm tofu in a frying pan and cook until vegetables are soft. Add firm tofu and chop and stir into vegetables. Add salsa on top.

## Oatmeal

Use thick-cut, steel-cut, or gluten-free oats and cook with filtered or spring water following directions. For each cup of oatmeal use ½ cup vanilla protein powder. Robb's is a great choice, which is sweetened with stevia. After oatmeal is cooked but protein powder in a bowl and mix with a small amount of water, non-fat or low-fat milk, or unsweetened vanilla almond milk to make powder into a thick liquid. Mix into oatmeal and add stevia and cinnamon. Spoon into a bowl and add fresh blueberries or peeled chopped apples and slivered almonds or chopped walnuts. (When traveling bring a baggie of dried dates and slivered almonds or chopped walnuts and stevia packets to use on oatmeal.)

## Cole Slaw

- Cabbage, chopped
- 1 carrot, shredded
- 1 clove garlic, crushed
- 1 tsp onion powder
- 1 tsp garlic pepper seasoning
- ½ T olive oil mayo or light mayo
- 2 T seasoned rice vinegar or apple cider vinegar

Add cabbage and carrot to large bowl. Add in all seasonings and mix well. Chill slaw before serving. (This can be made without any mayonnaise, if you prefer. Just add more rice vinegar for moisture.

## Deviled Eggs

- 6 eggs
- Dijon or yellow mustard to taste
- 1 tsp organic relish

Hard boil the eggs, then remove from heat and cool. Remove the shells and cut eggs in half. Place the yolks into a small bowl. Add mustard and relish and stir well. Scoop mixture into whites of eggs.

## Spinach Salad

- Fresh spinach
- 3 eggs, hard-boiled
- Cherry tomatoes, halved
- Balsamic vinegar

Place clean spinach in a bowl and add hard-boiled eggs and cherry tomato halves. Sprinkle with balsamic vinegar. Serve.

## SHRIMP SALAD

- Fresh Romaine lettuce, torn into small pieces
- 3-6 eggs, hard-boiled
- Tomatoes, chopped
- Avocado, diced

Light organic vinaigrette, homemade or organic cocktail sauce (no HFCS), or balsamic vinegar

Wash Romaine, tear into small pieces, and place into large bowl. Add 3-6 hard-boiled eggs, chopped tomatoes, and diced avocado. Add vinaigrette, cocktail sauce, or balsamic vinegar. Serve cold.

## VEGGIE & RICE SALAD

- Romaine lettuce, chopped
- Fresh spinach
- Tomato, chopped
- Avocado, sliced
- Garbanzo beans
- Kidney beans
- Pickled beets
- Red cabbage, chopped
- Broccoli, chopped
- Cauliflower, chopped
- Brown rice, cooked

Light organic vinaigrette or balsamic vinegar seasoned with rice vinegar

Prepare all the ingredients and place into a large bowl. Add brown rice. Top with vinaigrette or seasoned balsamic vinegar. (This salad has so many flavors, try eating it without any dressing. Taste all the flavors of real food!)

## BURRITO

Chop ground turkey breast in frying pan and cook until brown. Add organic vegetarian refried beans or black beans. Can also add leftover brown rice and steamed vegetables. Heat a large Ezekiel or Alvarado Street tortilla. Add shredded romaine lettuce and salsa. Wrap and eat. (Chop some fresh spinach and cilantro with lettuce for more nutrients and flavor.)

## TACO SALAD

Chop ground turkey breast in a frying pan and add taco spice or salt-free taco spice. Heat steamed mixed vegetables or cook frozen vegetables and add to turkey. Place ground turkey on top of shell and add salsa. (Can also add chopped avocado and tomato.)

## TACO SALAD WITH BEANS

Prepare same as above or use leftover ground turkey. Heat in frying pan and add organic vegetarian refried beans or black beans. Add vegetables and salsa.

Chop ground turkey in frying pan and add taco spices or salt-free taco spice and cook until browned. Add salsa and mixed vegetables (frozen or steamed) and heat until hot. Heat a small Ezekiel tortilla shell in frying pan and put taco meat in the shell.

## TRACY'S CHICKEN SOUP

Buy a whole organic chicken and remove all the skin, rinse inside and out (or use neck and back bones and two chicken breasts and remove skin). Put in a large pot of filtered or spring water to cover all the chicken about ¾ to the top. Chop one large brown onion and a whole head of celery, excluding the leafy part. Add two bay leaves, 3 cloves of peeled chopped garlic, and a bunch of parsley tied together with wax-free dental floss. Bring to boil and simmer until all the chicken is fully cooked and the vegetables are tender. Remove parsley and chicken bones. Make sure to get all the small bones out of the soup using a strainer spoon. Take meat off the bones and tear into small pieces and put back into the soup. Skim the fat off the top of the soup with a large cold tablespoon. Add 8 to 10 chopped carrots and cook until tender.

## TRACY'S VEGETARIAN SPLIT PEA SOUP

Same as above, but add 4 or 5 slices of turkey bacon for flavor. It can be removed after peas are cooked or chopped up and eaten with soup.

## TRACY'S BAKED BEANS

Soak rinsed navy beans or small white beans in a pot of water for one hour. Rinse and put in large pot with filtered or spring water to cover beans. Add 6 slices of turkey bacon, 3 spoons of xylitol, 1 tablespoon of brown sugar and 1 tablespoon of molasses. (Brown sugar and molasses are for color and can be omitted for sugar-free beans.) Simmer until beans are soft. Add salt to taste and more sweetener, if desired.

## TRACY'S VEGETARIAN BAKED BEANS

Same as above, but leave out the bacon and use Bragg's Liquid Amino Acids and liquid smoke for flavor.

## ROASTED CHICKEN

Organic chicken with neck and skin removed. Using a cooking bag or just put in a roasting bag and cook. Chicken can be eaten with steamed vegetables and steamed yams. Leftovers can be used for chicken tacos, burritos, chicken sandwich, and chicken salad. Save carcass to make chicken soup. If you are going to use it within a few days, put it in a freezer bag and freeze until ready to use.

## ROASTED TURKEY

Buy organic turkey and remove giblets and neck; rinse inside and out. Place turkey in a roasting pan and follow cooking instructions. Using a cooking bag will cook the turkey faster. Cover top with foil so it does not burn. Take off foil the last 30 minutes. Remove skin from turkey before serving. Save carcass to make turkey soup or put in a freezer bag to make soup with at another time.

## TURKEY LEFTOVERS

- Turkey sandwich with turkey breast and cranberry sauce.
- Turkey breast, toasted Ezekiel bread, mustard, lettuce, and tomato.
- Turkey with Japanese yam and baked beans. Add mixed vegetables.
- Turkey Benedict–see recipe above.

- Turkey bowl–put ½ cup brown rice or mashed potatoes in a bowl with turkey breast, mixed vegetables, and a spoon of baked beans.
- Turkey pot pie–can be made with low-fat cream of chicken soup, mixed vegetables, and chopped turkey. Make a crust or buy one made with 100% whole grains and just eat the middle or leave the crust off.

# CHAPTER 19: WEEKLY MENUS

## MEALS FOR THE WEEK

Every morning upon waking, drink a full glass of water with the juice of half a lemon. Have something to eat before your morning exercise. You will have more energy for you exercise if you are hydrated and have something to eat before you work out. Even if you just eat a banana and some peanut butter or some almonds. I keep almonds or raw trail mix in my gym bag in case I get hungry.

For people who exercise in the afternoon start your day with my healthy breakfast options. You may substitute any vegetables you like as long as they are non-starchy vegetables. Bread, grains, winter squash, yams, potatoes and pasta are starches. You may substitute something you like better but keep your starchy carbohydrates to one serving per meal.

If you get hungry in the afternoon you can take one of your starchy vegetables or grains and have it as a snack before dinner and not have a starch at dinner time. if you are trying to lose weight it is good to eat starchy carbohydrates during the day when you are more active.

One thing to keep in mind is when you eat more calories at one meal than your body is going to use up your body will store them as fat to be used later. The idea is to eat the majority of your food during the morning and afternoon when you are active.

All the meals in this two-week meal plan are just suggestions. You may want to substitute other types of protein or vegetables. The most important thing to remember is that I am giving you healthy meal options and suggesting portion control for those who want to lose weight. Learn to listen to your body and it will let you know what it needs.

If you hear a burger, fries and milkshake calling you are probably listening to an old message that needs to be erased from your head. Replace it with a turkey breast patty on Ezekiel toast with

Tracy's "unfries". This gives you a healthy version of what you may be craving that will satisfy the craving in a healthy way.

Eat breakfast every morning whether you work out or not. Skip the morning snack and go straight to breakfast. After a long night of fasting and rebuilding, your body needs nutrient dense foods and water.

## DAY 1

Snack Before Morning Exercise

- glass of water with juice of half a lemon
- Ezekiel toast with Better Than Peanut Butter or Almond butter lightly spread

Breakfast

- 3 egg whites scrambled with zucchini and broccoli
- 1 slice of Ezekiel sesame bread with Better than Peanut Butter and simple fruit lightly spread

Snack

- low fat cottage cheese (organic)
- sliced apples
- sprinkle of slivered almonds

Lunch

- Ezekiel bread
- tuna canned in water (drain), with unsweetened relish. (Make sure it does not have HFCS.)
- Romaine lettuce
- Tomato slice
- Cucumber slices

Snack

- Bowl of mixed fresh fruit and berries
- ½ cup plain Greek yogurt withstevia.

Dinner

- chicken breast
- half a Japanese yam
- cauliflower (steamed)
- Spinach salad with cucumber, broccoli slaw, or cabbage. (Use Balsamic, apple cider or rice vinegar that does not have HFCS.)

## DAY 2

Snack Before Exercise

- Glass of water with juice of half a lemon
- Ezekiel raisin toast with low-fat cottage cheese (sprinkle of cinnamon and stevia on top)

Breakfast

- 1 cup cooked steel cut oatmeal (add ½ scoop of Robb's egg white or whey protein mixed with water, almond milk or regular milk mixed into cooked oatmeal while hot)
- Sprinkle of cinnamon, stevia, slivered almonds and peeled apple chopped in small pieces, or dried chopped dates

Snack

- Half a large Japanese yam
- Low-fat string cheese

Lunch

- ½ large Ezekiel tortilla shell heated in frying pan
- Chicken breast cut in small pieces
- 1 - 2 tablespoons of organic vegetarian refried beans
- Spoon of low-fat cottage cheese (optional)
- Shredded lettuce
- Salsa

Snack

- 8-10 raw almonds
- ½ cup of organic low-fat plain Greek yogurt
- Blueberries (with or without stevia)

Dinner

- Salmon, broiled or cooked on stovetop
- Broccoli, steamed
- 1/2 - 1 cup brown rice, cooked without butter.
- Salad with romaine lettuce, red cabbage, garbanzo beans, and balsamic vinegar

## Day 3

Snack Before Exercise

- Ezekiel or Alvarado Street bread
- Almond cheese, chao cheese, or low-fat mozzarella cheese

Breakfast

- Ezekiel sesame toast
- 1 poached egg,
- Fresh oven-roasted turkey (free of hormones, antibiotics and nitrates)
- 1 slice of heart smart cheese or veggie cheese

Snack

- Small yam
- ½ cup of low-fat cottage (preferably organic)

Lunch

- Small Ezekiel tortilla shell heated on the stove

- 2 tablespoons of vegetarian black beans mixed with ½ cup of brown rice and salsa, topped with shredded or chopped romaine lettuce. (This can be eaten with or without a shell.)

Snack

- 2 brown rice cakes
- Almond butter (lightly spread on top)

Dinner

- Spinach salad with red cabbage, garbanzo beans, beets, avocado
- MahiMahi(baked, broiled, or cooked on stovetop without butter or oil)
- Any type of raw or steamed vegetable

## DAY 4

Snack before Exercise

- 100% rye bread
- Low-fat cottage cheese

Breakfast

- Ezekiel raisin bread dipped in egg whites and one whole egg for Tracy's French Toast. Dip bread into egg and then put in non-stick frying pan and cook on both sides. Sprinkle cinnamon and Stevia on top.
- Organic veggie patty (such as Amy's organic California-style veggie burger)

Snack

- Fruit smoothie with fresh or frozen strawberries and blueberries, ½ a banana, 1 scoop protein powder that does not have sugar, preservatives or artificial ingredients such as Robb's or other brand that uses stevia instead of sugar. Use vanilla or plain protein powder. Add almond milk, low fat milk or water plus ice cubes and blend to desired smoothness.

Lunch

- Salad with romaine lettuce, spinach, red cabbage, garbanzo beans, kidney beans, cherry tomatoes, beets and any other raw vegetables
- Top with ground turkey breast patty.
- Any type of mustard can be mixed with a small amount of organic ketchup to put on top.

Snack

- Medium yam
- Plain Greek yogurt with fresh blueberries and stevia

Dinner

- Grilled chicken breast with garlic powder and any salt-free seasoning
- Cauliflower mash
- Mixed vegetables
- Kabocha squash

## DAY 5

Snack before Exercise

- Ezekiel English muffin with Better Than Peanut Butter and Simple fruit

Breakfast

- Scrambles eggs ( 2 egg whites and one whole egg)
- Ezekiel English muffin, toasted.
- Fresh oven-roasted turkey (nitrate, antibiotic, and hormone free), heated. Cut thick slice and put on top of muffin, then add egg. (Either put the other half of the muffin on top or leave open faced.)

Snack

- ¼ cup of hummus
- Fresh raw vegetables
- 100% whole grain pretzels

Lunch

- Amy's Bean and Rice Burrito
- Amy's salsa or Muir Glen organic salsa

Snack

- Protein smoothie with plain Greek yogurt, 1 scoop protein powder, fresh berries and stevia. Blend with ice and ½ cup of spring or filtered water.

Dinner

- Salmon (grilled, broiled, or cooked on stove top)
- Salad with spinach, red cabbage, garbanzo beans, balsamic vinegar
- Broccoli and cauliflower, steamed
- ½ cup quinoa

## Day 6

Snack before Exercise

- Protein smoothie with fresh fruit, 1 scoop protein powder, almond milk, and yogurt with stevia.

Breakfast

- Steamed vegetables added to scrambled egg whites with one whole egg
- Yukon Gold potatoes cooked in microwave and cut into cubes. Put foil on cookie sheet and wipe with olive oil or olive oil spray and put potatoes on sheet. Sprinkle with garlic powder and salt-free seasoning. Put in oven on broil and cook them until they are brown. I call these Tracy's "Un-Fries." Cut them like French fries or home fries. (May use agave or organic ketchup.)

## DAY 7

Snack before Exercise

- Toast with almond cheese or
- Or banana with Better Than Peanut Butter

Breakfast

- Scrambled eggs (3 egg whites and one whole egg)
- Steamed veggies (whatever is left-over from you steamed vegetables or cook zucchini and mushrooms in a frying pan and add whipped eggs and cook).
- Slice of Ezekiel sesame bread, toasted, topped with almond butter and simple fruit spread lightly.

Snack

- ½ Japanese yam
- ½ cup low-fat organic cottage cheese

Lunch

- Salmon, poached or grilled
- Salad of spinach, romaine lettuce, tomatoes, and avocado. Top with balsamic vinegar

Snack

- Two lightly salted brown rice cakes with almond butter lightly spread

Dinner

- Whole wheat pasta
- chicken breast or shrimp, topped with crushed organic stewed tomatoes or fire roasted tomato sauce

Eat as many vegetables throughout the day as you wish. When you eat fruit try to combine it with protein or a fat such as 8 almonds. This will keep your blood sugar stable. Eating fruit alone is fine if you don't experience any dips in energy an hour or two later.

Substitute any type of protein as long as it is broiled, grilled, or cooked on the stovetop. If you choose to eat beef use it sparingly and only the leanest organic cuts. Use ground turkey breast instead of ground beef. To add moisture to ground turkey breast add a drizzle of organic barbeque sauce, agave ketchup or Bragg's Liquid amino acids and garlic powder. If you are going to use it for a Mexican dish add some organic salsa and salt-free taco seasoning.

## WEEK 2

### DAY 1

Snack before Exercise

- ¾ cup Millet Rice cereal
- Unsweetened vanilla almond milk or banana and raw almonds

Breakfast

- Steel cut oatmeal (add fresh blueberries or another type of berries and stevia)
- Smoothie with whey protein powder sweetened with stevia. Add raspberries, half a banana, unsweetened almond milk and ice then blend.

Snack

- Ezekiel raisin bread
- Low-fat organic cottage cheese, cinnamon, and stevia
- Fruit salad made with three types of seasonal fruit

Lunch

- Quinoa and brown rice on bed of Romaine lettuce, mixed steamed vegetables and tofu with light organic or homemade teriyaki sauce used sparingly. (Note that some people may prefer quinoa by itself or mixed with another grain.)

Snack

- Raw carrots, zucchini, broccoli and cauliflower with salsa or Tracy's bean and salsa dip

Dinner

- Tracy's Stuffed Acorn Squash
- Side salad with spinach, chopped tomatoes, ¼ avocado, and balsamic vinegar

## DAY 2

Snack before Exercise

- Ezekiel toast with Better than Peanut Butter and simple fruit lightly spread

Breakfast

- 1 poached egg
- 2 slices oven-roasted turkey breast, thick cut (hormone-, nitrate-, and antibiotic-free)
- Ezekiel English muffin, toasted with slice of veggie cheese
- Add fresh spinach and tomato for more nutrients (Use left-overs from last night's salad.)

Snack

- Hummus and raw vegetables of any type

Lunch

- ½ a cooked chicken breast
- 1-2 tablespoons of vegetarian refried pinto or black beans
- 1 tablespoon of salsa
- 1 small Ezekiel or Alvarado Street tortilla (heated to desired firmness)
- Serve with shredded Romaine lettuce and 1 tablespoon of low-fat cottage cheese (optional)

Snack

- Tracy's Cauliflower Pie
- Kabocha squash

Dinner

- Boneless skinless chicken breast (broiled or cooked in a pan)
- Slice of tomato with one slice of low fat mozzarella cheese. Bake in oven until cheese melts of gets warm

## Day 3

Snack before Exercise

- Ezekiel raisin toast
- Low-fat cottage cheese, cinnamon, and stevia

Breakfast

- 3 egg whites, scrambled
- ¼ avocado
- Ezekiel English muffin

Snack

- Plain Greek yogurt, low- or nonfat
- Fresh berries and stevia

Lunch

- Salmon, grilled or poached
- Salad with romaine lettuce, cherry tomatoes, and red cabbage
- Half a Japanese yam

Snack

- Broccoli and carrots, steamed (Bragg's Liquid Amino Acids for added flavor)
- ½ cup low-fat cottage cheese or low-fat string cheese

Dinner

- Veggie "unfry" with frozen mixed, Chinese, and Thai mixed vegetables, firm organic tofu with Bragg's Liquid Amino Acids

Day 4
Snack before Exercise

- 100% whole wheat crackers and Better Than Peanut Butter

Breakfast

- Oatmeal with protein powder, slivered almond, chopped apples, and stevia

Snack

- Japanese yam

Lunch

- 1 slice Ezekiel sesame bread
- chicken breast, grilled
- Mustard, lettuce, tomato, and cucumber

Snack

- 1 cup of Tracy's Vegetarian Split Pea soup with carrots

Dinner

- Scallops, grilled
- Asparagus
- Spinach salad with red cabbage and balsamic vinegar

## DAY 5

Snack before Exercise

- Ezekiel or Alvarado Street bread, toasted
- Almond butter

Breakfast

- Leftover oatmeal (heated up) with protein powder

- Fresh blueberries and stevia

Snack
½ cup of low-fat cottage cheese with chopped apple and slivered almonds
Lunch
Amy's Bean and Rice Burrito with salsa
Snack
Brown rice cakes (lightly salted) with Better Than Peanut Butter
Dinner

- Salmon, grilled or cooked on stovetop
- Broccoli and cauliflower, steamed
- Tracy's home "un-fries" made with Yukon Potatoes

## Day 6

Snack before Exercise

- protein shake with stevia and mixed berries

Breakfast

- Egg white scramble with fresh or frozen vegetables
- Ezekiel sesame toast and with almond butter

Snack

- Hardboiled egg
- 4 whole grain crackers

Lunch

- Salmon
- Brown rice
- Steamed broccoli

Snack

- Bread Pizza (low-fat cheese on Ezekiel toast with agave ketchup, garlic powder, and powdered oregano)

Dinner

- Ground turkey breast
- Mixed vegetables
- Salsa and 1 tablespoon of organic vegetarian refried beans. (Cut 2 bell peppers in half and remove seeds. Steam upside down until soft. Stuff with mixture.)

## Day 7

Snack before Exercise

- Ezekiel Sesame toast with almond cheese

Breakfast

- Tracy's home "un-fries" seasoned with garlic powder and garlic pepper
- Veggie egg white scramble
- Agave ketchup or salsa

Snack

- Fruit salad
- Plain Greek yogurt and stevia

Lunch

- Small Ezekiel shell
- Chicken breast, grilled
- black beans(Top with salsa and low fat cottage cheese, if desired)

Snack

- 2 brown rice cakes with simple fruit and Better Than Peanut butter
- Carrots and broccoli, raw or steamed

Dinner

- Brown rice sushi tuna and avocado, Hamachi sashimi and ginger and rice paper roll with shrimp or tofu. (Most organic food stores have a sushi bar where you can order or choose from what they already have made.)

This menu plan is only to give an example of what can be made for each meal and snack. As long as you stay within the guidelines of my healthy eating plan, mix and match whatever you want to make meals from and use leftovers to create different meals.

When choosing pasta make sure it is 100% whole grain and does not have any artificial ingredients or preservatives. Tomato sauce is easy to make if you buy organic tomato sauce, stewed tomatoes, and add Italian spices. Many of the sauces have artificial flavors, preservatives, or high fructose corn syrup and sugar. These can be avoided by making your own sauce. It does not have to cook all day or be a long drawn out process unless you have a special family recipe that you want to use.

I suggest making sure to remove any sugar or excess salt and use garlic powder and Italian herbs. Create your own new recipe for the family using healthy ingredients. Kids actually love chunky sauce and fusilli pasta which has a spiral shape. We call it curly pasta. It is fun for the kids and comes in 100% whole grain.

Cheese is something that many people like to eat, but it's high in cholesterol and saturated fat which can contribute to heart disease. I have given you cheese alternatives like Heart Healthy Cheese, Go Veggie Cheese, Almond Cheese, and Chao Cheese which are all non-dairy.

Using dairy products that are low or non-fat will cut down on the amount of saturated fat and cholesterol. Check with your doctor to see if you need to lose weight or for the guidelines for children if your children do not eat dairy products they may need to supplement with other foods to get the amount of calcium and protein children need for strong bones and teeth.

When choosing what to eat strive for a wide variety of fresh fruits and vegetables and healthy carbohydrates and lean protein. The meal plan I have provided is something that you can use as a guide to help you create meals that are healthy and nutrient dense. By simple cutting out fast food, processed food, and sugary treats you already have a great start toward improving your health. Making changes will be easy when you realize how much you will gain by eat healthy foods.

# ABOUT THE AUTHOR

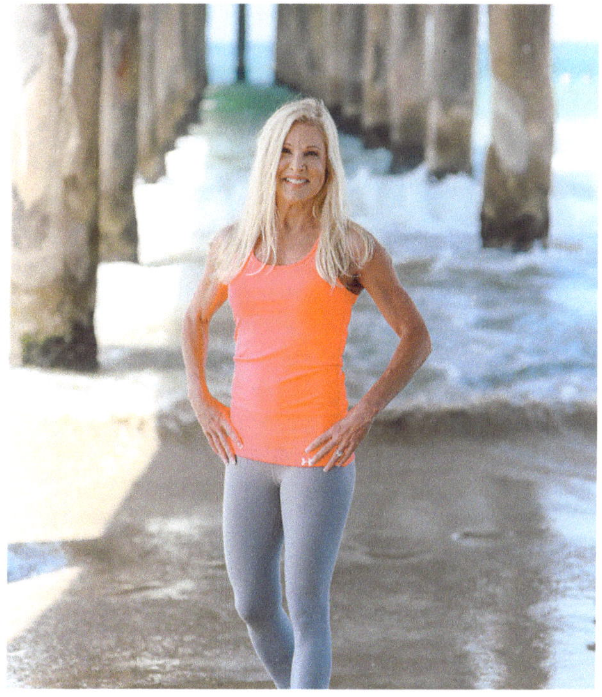

Tracy Dwyer attended Pepperdine University in Malibu and has a Bachelor of Arts Degree in Film and Television from Loyola Marymount University in Los Angeles, California. She started two successful businesses, one in Los Angeles and one in San Jose, California. Tracy and her son, Justin Rowland, moved to San Jose, California, where she worked for a television station as a videographer for the news as well as working for televised special events, church services, city council meetings, and television programs.

Tracy also has been seen in front of the camera as an actor. She has appeared in several television series such as *Nash Bridges* and the movie, *Patch Adams*, as well as appearing in many local and national commercials. She is a lifetime practitioner and acolyte of nutrition and living a healthy happy life. She wrote this book to share her voluminous knowledge.

She met her husband, Gerald Dwyer, while living in Campbell, California. He was an officer in the U.S. military. After 9-11 he was called to take command of a Chinook helicopter unit at Fort Hood, Texas. It was there that Tracy became the head of The Family Readiness Group to prepare and assist the families of the soldiers who were about to be deployed. She also became active in the Officers Wives' Club and the New Comers Club in Belton, Texas. They lived in Morgan's Point Resort during the two-year command and then were sent to serve at Redstone Arsenal in Huntsville, Alabama.

Tracy Dwyer gained a great deal of knowledge in the field of nutrition and has made it her mission to help people learn how to make healthy eating and exercise a priority in their lives. It has been more than two decades since her unlikely diagnosis of colon cancer at a very young age and she remained healthy with no recurrence of cancer due to her healthy eating and exercise lifestyle as reflected in this book. As a very young colon cancer survivor she became passionate in spreading awareness about this cancer and the fact that it can, indeed, strike young people. To that end she worked closely with the American Cancer Society creating Public Service Announcements on television and through her motivational speaking engagements.

For more information or to invite Tracy to speak, you may contact her at: tracydwyer.com

www.ingramcontent.com/pod-product-compliance
Lightning Source LLC
Chambersburg PA
CBHW040932030426
42336CB00001B/2
* 9 7 8 1 4 9 9 9 0 5 2 4 3 *